THERAPY OUTCOME MEASURES (TOM)
Speech and Language Therapy

TECHNICAL MANUAL

THERAPY OUTCOME MEASURES (TOM)
Speech and Language Therapy

TECHNICAL MANUAL

Professor Pam Enderby Ph.D., M.Sc., F.C.S.L.T., M.B.E.

with

Alexandra John M.Sc., M.C.S.L.T.

The University of Sheffield
Community Sciences Centre
Northern General Hospital
Sheffield, England

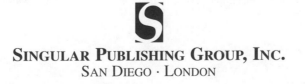

SINGULAR PUBLISHING GROUP, INC.
SAN DIEGO · LONDON

Order # 1578
Therapy Outcome Measures
Must Include: User's Manual, Technical Manual, A set of 10 Cards.
The ISBN # for the whole set is: 1-56593-494-6.

Singular Publishing Group, Inc.
401 West A Street, Suite 325
San Diego, California 92101-7904

19 Compton Terrace
London N1 2UN, U.K.

e-mail: singpub@mail.cerfnet.com
Website: http://www.singpub.com

© 1997 by Singular Publishing Group, Inc.

Typeset in 11/14 Times by So Cal Graphics
Printed in the United States of America by McNaughton & Gunn

ISBN: 1-56593-807-0

ACKNOWLEDGMENTS

1. This work was supported by a grant from the Department of Health and the Underwood Trust. We are grateful for their financial assistance, stimulating interest, and constructive comments.
2. Many therapists have volunteered to take part in the project. The mature willingness of the profession to investigate their effectiveness, to wish to improve the quality of their services, and to take on even more work was admirable and much appreciated.
3. We acknowledge the invaluable assistance of the Research Team at the Speech and Language Therapy Research Unit and particularly that of Mrs. Sally McConnell in all aspects of this project. We appreciate the specific assistance of Dr. Brian Petheram and Mrs. Marina Sloan who gave assistance with many practical aspects of the project implementation.
4. We are grateful to the following sites for their participation, collaboration, and assistance with this project:

   Frenchay Health Care Trust
   Phoenix NHS Trust
   Royal Gloucester and Severn NHS Trust
   East Wiltshire Health Trust
   Hammersmith Hospital
   St Mary and St Charles Hospital Trust
   East Gloucester
   East Berkshire

The views expressed in this report are those of the authors and not necessarily of the Department of Health.

CONTENTS

LIST OF TABLES

EXECUTIVE SUMMARY

Speech and language therapists have many standardized assessments to assist them in diagnosing patients and monitoring change. The majority of these tools relate to specific aspects of speech and language impairment and were developed for use with particular client groups. The current tools do not lend themselves easily to outcome studies as most are lengthy and complicated and are not designed to capture needs and change in domains associated with the broad goals of therapy. The project reported here developed and standardized a common approach which aims to capture information related not only to the impairment, but also to disability, handicap, and wellbeing—all areas therapists attempt to influence in the rehabilitation of persons with communication disorders.

This study tested the approach in eight districts and gathered information on more than 1,000 patients in order to examine its practicality, reliability, validity, acceptability, and sensitivity. The tool is now in a format that can act as a stable platform for further developments (e.g., development of a similar approach for users and caregivers and other professionals) and evaluations of therapy outcomes.

The approach is being used to develop similar measures suitable for use by occupational therapists, physiotherapists, and podiatrists, and trials are underway. Additionally, we are piloting a similar approach for users and caregivers to monitor outcomes.

Introduction

Recent radical changes in health service delivery have increased the pressure on all service providers to examine their methods for reporting results relating to the impact of health services (Wilkin, Hallam, & Doggett, 1992). There is a greater awareness of the disparity of health care, widely differing costs, and concerns about demonstrable effectiveness. Information reflecting the effects of treatment is essential in order to modify methods of provision, influence purchasing patterns, and assist in monitoring contracts along with harnessing efforts to improve care (Ware, 1991). Hence, professionals are becoming more conscious of their social as well as clinical responsibility to account for the value and benefits of interventions.

The importance of basing health care on a firm knowledge base to improve cost-effectiveness and efficiency is highly laudable. However, moving toward gathering information in a formal and reliable way that will assist in clarifying health gain is considerably more complex than has been recognized. Thus, there remains a tendency to equate the outcome of an activity with the rate at which patients are being referred or discharged rather than determining the impact of particular care packages on an individual's health (Hopkins, 1993).

"Purchasers are not indifferent to the question of quality but they are stymied by the 'current state of the art' in quality measurement" (Health Care Advisory Board, 1994, p. 32); this is due both to clinical and technological limitations and different views regarding what constitutes quality. Meaningful data are hard to find and even harder to decipher.

Outcome measurement is complex because it is difficult to define the effects of care and frequently there is little agreement regarding what health programs are endeavoring to achieve with different client groups. For example, with a patient with progressive neurological disease, it may be more appropriate for a clinician to be concerned with appropriate pain management and the assurance that death is going to be handled appropriately rather than with a "cure."

Most outcome measures have concentrated on negative outcomes, such as the reduction of morbidity and mortality, and have failed to reflect the quality of care received by the majority of patients who are influenced positively by their treatment. Further difficulties arise when one examines the complexity of what health services try to deliver. Health care programs frequently include aspects such as prevention of disease, information for patients and relatives, supporting, counseling, and managing secondary complications. Thus, the measures of outcome that are used currently may be seen as reflecting a simplistic view of the aims of the health intervention.

Informing investment for health care on objective evidence has led to a greater reliance on published research. In most medical and rehabilitation fields, there is a limited amount of conclusive research that can be used alone to inform practice. Frequently, research attracts specific cohorts of patients that do not reflect the range of difficulties requiring health service involvement in a wide range of settings. Furthermore, although research is essential, purchasers and managers have difficulty using research as a benchmark for their own practices if there are no methods to continually monitor the performance of patients within localities on a regular basis for comparative purposes.

Many health status/outcome and assessment scales purport to provide objective data on populations and specific subgroups. Donovan, Frankel, and Eyles, (1993) gave an overview of health status measures divided into six cateogries:

1. **General Health Measures.** These provide global profiles of health, including wellbeing, function, and social and emotional health; for example, General Health Questionnaires

(Goldberg & Hillier, 1979), Nottingham Health Profile (Hunt & McEwan, 1980), Medical Outcomes study instrument SF36 (Riesenberg & Glass, 1989).

2. **Measures of Physical Function.** These reflect the level of physical impairment and disability within general populations; for example, Lambeth Disability Screening Questionnaire (Patrick et al., 1981) or for specific groups; for example, a unified Activities of Daily Living (ADL) evaluation form (Donaldson, Vagner, & Gresham, 1973). These assess functions such as dressing, mobility, and self-care.

3. **Pain Measures.** Instruments that are generally used with specific client groups and reflect the intensity/duration of pain; for example, McGill Pain Questionnaire (Melzack, 1983), the Visual Analogue Scale (Scott & Huskisson, 1979).

4. **Social Health Measures.** The Social Health Battery (Williams, Ware, & Donald, 1981) and similar batteries assess the strength of people's social support mechanisms, and networks.

5. **Quality of Life Measures.** The Four Single Items of Wellbeing (Andrews & Crandall, 1976) and the Quality of Life Index (Spitzer, Dobson, & Hall, 1981) measure the elusive "satisfaction of individuals with life."

6. **Specific Disease Measures.** These measures assess issues relevant to particular client groups in order to establish the impact and/or severity of conditions; for example, the Arthritis Impact Measurement Scale (Meenan, Gertman, & Mason, 1980), The Frenchay Dysarthria Assessment (Enderby, 1981).

These are a few of the plethora of different tools and approaches used to monitor the performance of patients who have different diseases/health difficulties and who are receiving input from numerous health professionals. However, collecting, pooling, and comparing these data are difficult and end up being less than informative for those who wish to make decisions. Traditional clinical indicators used in health research and outcome measurement have several major shortcomings: They tend to focus on rare negative outcomes and omit the degrees of benefit of certain treatments. Furthermore, other traditional measures focus on biological outcomes, for example, reductions in spasticity, infections, or amputations. It is well-known that health is considerably more to an individual than the reduction of disease alone. "Health is a slippery concept" (Anderson, Sullivan, & Usherwood, 1990, p. 205), a complex combination of lack of illness, wellbeing, control over life, and autonomy.

Despite considerable work on devising and validating impairment scales (Ebrahim, Nouri, & Barer, 1985; Wade 1992), their use in the clinic and in clinical trials has sometimes failed to reflect improvement where clinical judgment and other evidence suggests that therapy has been beneficial (Harewood et al., 1994). Most studies on the efficacy of different nursing and therapy professions have used measures of impairment; for example, the accuracy of articulation, muscle power, or range of movement. However, examination of what nursing and therapy try to achieve demonstrates that modifying impairment is only one component of the therapeutic target (Enderby, 1992). Thus, the primary goal of health care for many patients, particularly those with long-term chronic conditions, is to maximize function in everyday life and to achieve the highest level of wellbeing (Stewart et al., 1989).

The work presented here was stimulated by the desire to have a single simple measure that could reflect the status of an individual more broadly than is possible with other assessment procedures; the degree of "disorder" (i.e., impairment), the everyday limitations in function (i.e., disability), and the social consequences (i.e., handicap). Previously, therapists had to turn to different tools if they wished to assess the patient holistically. This often caused difficulties as the various tools are not designed to dovetail and may give different weightings to different components.

Speech and language therapists frequently aim to improve the communication skills of patients (despite the specific deficit), increase morale, overcome withdrawal, improve knowledge about the disorder, support caregivers, and many other aspects that are considered to lead to an appropriate holistic approach to a person requiring this health intervention.

Consideration was given as to whether it would be appropriate to adapt other scales (e.g., Functional Independence Measure/Functional Activity Measure [FIM/FAM], Functional Limitation Profile [FLP]), which do contain elements related to communication. Although adapting tools may be preferable in some ways, this was not considered appropriate for our purposes, as the concepts related to communication in those tools were too limited and could not be adapted to reflect sufficient aspects relevant to the various disorders of communication. Furthermore, the measures did not relate to the goals frequently set by therapists and therefore may not reflect outcome to treatment.

The starting point of outcome measurement should be a greater understanding about what is to be achieved within a health care program. Retrospective studies of outcome in child language disorders, although principally assessing the language impairment, have documented the effects of language impairment on the functional communication and social and emotional development of the child. It has been observed that young children who have difficulty communicating verbally experience frustration and may, over time, become socially isolated. Therapists will try to reduce this effect (Bishop & Edmundson, 1987; Byers, Brown, & Edwards, 1989; Cantwell & Baker, 1987; Crowley, 1992). It has been considered good practice, based on research evidence, that therapy for stammering should include an emphasis on changing attitudes along with increasing fluency; similarly, speech and language therapy for dysphasia/aphasia includes elements of supporting and educating the relatives in communication strategies along with specific treatment to improve word usage. These bring a diverse range of goals which need to be assessed in order to judge the real benefits of treatment. It is obvious that measuring linguistic features alone would not be enough, and this underlines the need to develop multidimensional outcome measures in order that the effect of different health services in all aspects of management can be reflected.

Assessment of treatment outcomes is complicated by the multiplicity of objectives in most treatment programs which are not readily measured, as they involve goals other than those assessed by the standard procedures for assessing impairment.

Health service authorities have been charged with the responsibility to purchase a pattern of health care provisions that accords with the needs of the local population (Department of Health, 1989). This stimulated a resurgence of interest in surveying population needs along with the efforts to establish effectiveness of services. The measures outlined by Donovan, Frankel, and Eyles (1993) have occasionally been used to survey health needs as well as to measure effectiveness. However, most measures were originally designed for one or the other purpose and do not necessarily transfer readily. Even when contained in the field of establishing health needs, Donovan et al. argued that they may be less effective than hoped, as the level of generalizable characteristics of health status measures makes their interpretation difficult and possibly inadequate to support purchasing decisions, as it is not possible to map general measures of pain, mobility, or distress to the requirements for specific services. We would suggest that this places an even higher demand on the need for service outcome data.

In most specialties there are wide variations in clinical practice with limited agreement as to the most effective treatment, limited criteria to indicate the appropriate level of intervention, and a lack of information that the intervention itself is justified. The small amount of research in some fields only fuels debate rather than giving answers that would help to define best practice. Thus, there is a continued tendency to equate the outcome of activity with process measures, such as throughput and activity levels, rather than determining the effect of the care package in its totality, which is the aim of the project reported here.

CHAPTER 1

International Classification of Impairment, Disability, and Handicap

If health care processes are to be evaluated, they must be goal orientated because the appraisal is concerned with the extent to which goals are obtained. The prime requirement is for clearly specified outcome goals and this would permit a study of the extent to which these outcome goals are met, the effectiveness of the particular health care process; the inputs necessary to obtain this, the efficiency of the process; and its availability and uptake (Cochrane, 1972).

In response to this, the World Health Organization (WHO) emphasized that outcomes should be related to goals. However, it was noted that the simplest requirement of the health care system is that "some beneficial change in the individual's situation or status should result from the contact with that system." If there is no change, then the value of a given health care process should be seriously open to question. Thus, more than a decade ago, the challenge was thrown down to find a means of describing the status of an individual in such a way that changes could be appropriately recorded (Wood & Badley, 1978).

The realization that health care systems were attempting to have a broader impact than the reduction and prevention of disease alone necessitated the development of a language that could reflect an extension to the sequence of events underlying illness-related phenomena. Wood & Badley (1978) and Wood (1980) suggested the following profile:

disease → impairment → disability → handicap.

The definitions accorded to the terms *impairment*, *disability*, and *handicap* are summarized in **Table 1–1**.

Table 1–1. World Health Organization's Definitions of impairment, disability, and handicap.

IMPAIRMENT	Dysfunction resulting from pathological changes in system
DISABILITY	Consequence of impairment in terms of functional performance (disturbance at level of person)
HANDICAP	Disadvantages experienced by the individual as a result of impairment and disabilities; reflects interaction with and adaptation to the individual's surroundings

Although the International Classification of Impairment, Disability, and Handicap (ICIDH) classification is being revised[1] it appears unlikely that the changes will have a substantial effect on the work presented here. The details of the classification have not been used in this study, which is confined to the top-level headings of impairment, disability, and handicap. The second revision meeting in Washington D.C. 1993 endorsed the domain of impairment as "body/organ," the domain of disability as "person," and the domain of handicap as largely "social," thus, the concepts will remain the same.

This form of classification allows one to reflect on the different impacts of illness on an individual. For example, some conditions will "impair" slightly but cause severe "disability"

[1]A revision of the International Classification of Impairment, Disability, and Handicap officially commenced in 1993 and was coordinated by the WCC WHO Collaborating Centre, Nationale Road voor de Volksgezondheid, P.O. Box 7100, 2701 AC Zoetmeer, Netherlands.

and "handicap," whereas others may show major "impairment" but limited "disability" and "handicap."

Studies have indicated poor correlations between the impairments, disabilities, and handicaps in some individuals from particular client groups. For example, in heart failure there may be no relation between cardiac output (impairment), treadmill exercise tolerance and timed walking tests (disabilities), and social activity (handicap) (Cowley et al., 1991). This lack of direct relationship between impairment, disability, and handicap also applies in chronic airway disease (Williams & Bury, 1989). From the patient's point of view, impairment may be of less importance than the restrictions placed on everyday life.

THE VALUE OF INTERNATIONAL CLASSIFICATION OF IMPAIRMENT, DISABILITY, AND HANDICAP TO THE THERAPY PROFESSIONS

The language used by professionals when assisting those with different health difficulties is, at present, diverse—even within one profession the descriptions of the disorders, the treatment methods, and the goals may be phrased in such different ways that communication is difficult. The use of the ICIDH definitions allows therapists to communicate more effectively with each other and with their managers. It also facilitates reflection of the different domains of the treatment which would be different according to the different client groups served. There has been an increasing clamor for the development of functional assessments, and some authors have even called for deficit measures (impairment) to be abandoned, particularly when evaluating rehabilitation (Blomert, 1990; Haley, Coster, & Ludlow, 1991). In actuality these are probably calls for the field to be redressed and balanced since "impairment scales" abound. This study is based on the beliefs that each domain needs to be given weight and be included when assessing.

INVESTIGATING WHETHER THE WHO CLASSIFICATION WOULD ASSIST IN IDENTIFYING THERAPY GOALS

A study of outcome measurement must essentially start with a full understanding of what a particular service is trying to achieve. This can then act as the benchmark for determining whether the stated goals have been achieved (Langton & Hewer, 1990). According to many authorities, speech and language therapy aims to:

- improve/remediate the underlying impairment to communication; for example, treat auditory attention deficits, phonological disorders, syntactic, semantic, or pragmatic disorders;
- extend functional communication; for example, by teaching signing systems, use of communication aids, or facilitated intelligibility;
- develop strategies to overcome the personal and social disadvantages of the deficit;
- support the patient and caregivers during the adjustment phase (Royal College of Speech and Language Therapists, 1996; Sarno, 1993, Wertz, 1983, 1987, 1993).

To establish whether the WHO classification would be appropriate for consideration for development as a model for outcomes, the notes from 300 cases receiving speech and language therapy were examined. The goals in these cases were identified, and a large majority could be included under the groupings of impairment, disability, and handicap. However, there were no client groups that did not have goals attributed to all of these sections. There was one group of goals identified by speech and language therapists that were difficult to mesh with this classification, those relating to the emotional wellbeing of clients and their families. Therapists frequently try to reduce anxiety, depression, anger, fear, and improve emotional control and coping strategies. Because so many goals were identified in this area, it was felt important to extend the classification by adding the heading of "**distress/wellbeing**" for the purposes of this study. The importance of addressing emotional aspects in health care was identified by Rosser (1976), and at that time he and his colleagues suggested this as a measurement of outcome.

Many treatises on the effectiveness of health service provision, rehabilitation, and outcome dwell on the importance of "quality of life." Although this term has become increasingly fashionable, it has not been defined (McKenna, Hunt, & Tennant, 1993). Therapists feel strongly that they contribute to improving the elusive *je ne sais quoi*. In this study we have avoided the use of the term "quality of life" as it means different things to different people. However, the essentials of this concept are probably captured in the domains of handicap and distress. Interestingly, no goals specifying "improving quality of life" were found in the case notes but goals to do with "improving self-esteem," "improving personal autonomy" (handicaps), "teaching coping strategies to reduce fear," and "helping the person to come to terms with (distress)" were mentioned frequently.

Therapists commonly regard "disease" as a psychophysiological process that limits the person's coping abilities; coping being the adaption under existential threat/stress (Fugl-Meyer, Branholm, & Fugl-Meyer, 1991). This belief underlies one of the aims of rehabilitation, which is to mobilize the resources of individuals so that, by having realistic goals, they may achieve optimal life satisfaction. McCrae and Costa, (1986) supported this philosophy, as they found that individuals who used effective coping strategies reported higher subsequent life satisfaction. These authors, along with many others (e.g. Frattali 1991; Stephen & Hetu, 1992; Whiteneck et al., 1992), support the ICIDH classification as one that can reflect the complexity of the challenges in rehabilitation (Stephen & Hetu, 1992).

CHAPTER 2

Development of the Outcome Scales

Eight pilot sites were recruited for the study and each pilot site assisted with the development of measures related to impairment, disability, handicap, and distress/wellbeing. These were done independently so that comparisons with regard to the validity and reliability could be made at a later stage.

Each pilot site was asked to identify key client groups with which their service was actively engaged, and with which they wished to develop individual scales. Table 2–1 identifies the pilot sites and the primary client groups selected for study purposes.

Table 2–1. Pilot sites and primary client groups.

Site	Number of Therapists Involved	Primary Client Groups Covered
Site 1. Acute Hospital and Community Trust	20	Fluency disorders, Dysphonia, Dysphasia/Aphasia, Dysarthria, Dysphagia, Learning difficulty, Developmental speech and language disorders, Hearing impairment
Site 2. Learning Disability Trust	22	Developmental language disorders, Learning disability/Mental retardation, Phonology
Site 3. Acute, Community, and Learning Disability Trust	32	Fluency disorders, Dysphonia, Dysphasia/Aphasia Developmental language disorders, Learning disability/Mental retardation, Phonology
Site 4. Acute, Community, and Learning Disability Trust	15	Fluency disorders, Dysphonia, Dysphagia, Developmental speech and language disorders, Learning disability/Mental Retardation
Site 5. Acute Hospital Trust	4	Dysphasia/Aphasia
Site 6. Acute, Community, and Learning Disability Trust	5	Dysphonia, Dysphasia/Aphasia, Dysphagia, Developmental speech and language disorders, Learning disability/Mental Retardation
Site 7. Community and Learning Disability Trust	20	Fluency disorders, Dysphonia, Dysphasia/Aphasia, Dysphagia, Learning disability/Mental retardation, Developmental language disorders, Phonology
Site 8. Community Trust	14	Fluency disorders, Developmental speech and language disorders, Learning disability/Mental Retardation, Dysphagia,
Total Number of Therapists Involved	132	

A training period of 3 hours was conducted in each pilot site. The initial training contained the following topics:

- Necessity for outcome measures
- What are outcome measures?
- What do we try and achieve in speech and language therapy?
- WHO classification
- Methods of developing scales
- Core scale concepts

SCALE DEVELOPMENT

Following initial training, each group was involved in developing 0–5 scales related to each domain. To assist the therapists in developing comparable scales, some restrictions were placed on them. These were as follows:

- The scales were from 0 to 5, with zero being the most severe.
- The concepts relating to each point on the scale tallied with those in the core scale (see Appendix A). This was to ensure comparability and uniformity.
- The therapists were asked to give as many descriptors as possible that would assist them to rate a patient appropriately within their specific client group. They were encouraged to define and specify what they meant by "severe," "moderate," "mild," "occasional," and "frequent."
- Each descriptor was not mutually inclusive, thus therapists were asked to give different descriptors within the same grade but which may not occur with the same patient; for example, a person may be totally deaf and this might be judged as the same severity as a patient with a complete auditory agnosia or receptive disorder.

How Many Points on the Scale?

The number of points on any measurement scale must be considered carefully. It is likely that a smaller number of points on the scale will improve its reliability; however, an increased number of points on the scale can produce a more sensitive and reflective measure. Work by others has indicated that scales with between 9 and 12 points often allow for both reliability and sensitivity (Nishisato & Tori, 1970; Streiner & Norman, 1989).

Although the scale is overtly 6 points, patients can be graded with half points, thus expanding the scale to 11 points in actuality. Therapists may grade patients using .5 to identify that they were slightly better or worse than a particular descriptor.

OUTCOME SCALES PRODUCED BY PILOT SITES

The outcome scales produced independently by the pilot sites had remarkable similarity, not only in the concepts, but also in the words used. Additionally, the scales for different client groups showed some similarities, particularly in the area of disability, handicap, and wellbeing. See Appendix B for examples of four scales produced for dysphasia/aphasia.

At a later stage in the project, these scales were amalgamated to form an agreed-on set. For the purposes of this pilot study, each district used the scales that they had developed independently. These were scrutinized by the researchers to ensure that the concepts of each domain were appropriate.

USER INVOLVEMENT

A method to capture the views of patients and (where appropriate) relatives regarding the outcome of therapy was challenging and not dealt with in as much depth as we would have liked (See "Future Requirements to Extend this Work," Appendix N). Initially, a 5-point scale was devised for use at the end of an episode of care to express the degree of concordance between patient/relative/therapist views of progress during treatment (Enderby, 1992; see Table 2–2).

Table 2–2. Initial agreement score.

1.	No change in view of patient/caregiver and professional.
2.	No change in view of patient/caregiver or professional.
3.	Change, but not as much as expected by patient/caregiver and professional.
4.	Change, but not as much as expected by patient/caregiver or professional.
5.	Change in line with expectations of patient/carer and professional.

A trial using this scale, which was hoped to assist with the interpretation and validity of the outcome scores, soon demonstrated that only 3 points were used. Additionally, the scale was confusing the concepts of "change" with "consensus"; it was thus reduced to 3 points reflecting the degree of consensus, see Table 2–3.

Table 2–3. Agreement score.

1.	Professional/client/caregiver do not agree on outcome.
2.	Professional/client/caregiver do not agree equally on outcome.
3.	Professional/client/caregiver agree on outcome in all domains.

Note. Agreement relates to agreed view even when there is no change in any domain; that is, client, caregiver or professional may have total agreement that nothing has changed.

PREDICTION OF OUTCOME

To set goals for therapy, therapists will frequently predict which aspects will change. They may predict change on tasks they are specifically targeting in therapy, related areas that they judge will be spontaneously improving, or in areas that may be enhanced as a secondary gain to the specific treatment. Although this aspect of the work could not be pursued due to time constraints, the data collection and software mechanisms were put in place to allow for this to be explored later.

USER GUIDELINES

The guidelines available in the accompanying user's manual assist the therapist in the practical management of scoring a patient. In summary, they specify that the therapist should:

1. enter the presenting scores for IDHW-coded A for admission;
2. enter a score coded I for any intermediate score, for example, when there is a new episode of care or a change in provision;
3. enter the final score-coded F for final.

Scores for separate episodes of care can be entered on the same form for an individual patient, see Figure 2–1. The notes to assist users in the project are found in Appendix C. The operational user's manual gives more detail regarding mechanisms of scoring.

SAMPLE

OUTCOME MEASURES CLIENT DETAIL
SPEECH AND LANGUAGE THERAPY

> **(1)** Patient Name or Identifying Code Number
> *James Bond 007*

(2) Therapy Profession   *SPEECH*
(Speech, Physio, Chiropody, Diet, O.T.)

(3) Service Provider   *ST. ELSEWHERES*

Patient Details

(4) Age   *34*   (Years)   **(5) Duration of Treatment**   *6*   (Months)   **(6) No. of Contacts**   *21*

(7) Locality   Check appropriate box

☐ Inpatient

☑ Outpatient

☐ Community

(8) Caregiver   *SPOUSE*
(Spouse, Mother, etc.)

(9) Client Care Group   Check appropriate box appropriate box Please tick one only

☐ Child

☑ Adult   *3*   *C*

(10) Etiology Code
(See overleaf for codes)

(11) Communication Code 1
(See overleaf for codes)

4

Communication Code 2
(as above)

6

(12) Ratings

Code*	(13) Impairment Imp1	Imp2	Disability	Handicap	(14) Wellbeing/Director Patient	Caregiver	Agreement	Date of Rating
A	1	3	2	3	3	2	NA	12/06/95
I	3	3	3.5	4	4	3	2	06/09/95
F	3.5	3	4	4	4	4	3	08/09/95

* A = Admission, I = Intermediate, F = Final.

(15) Comments _____

Note: You may wish to adapt this data collection form to suit your existing patient data system.

Figure 2–1. Example of completed data collection form.

CHAPTER 3

Pilot Study Data Collection

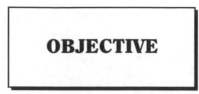

OBJECTIVE

The main aim of the pilot study was to establish whether therapists found this approach to be usable, practical, and valid.

Additionally, comments on each patient's profile were collected to establish which aspects of change were less adequately accommodated.

PROCEDURE

Each of the eight pilot districts was asked to gather outcome data on patients currently receiving treatment. Unfortunately the data collection period was short (3–5 months) and this necessitated the therapist recording the pretreatment score based on reflection and their own clinical records. This, of course, is less than adequate and is likely to have compromised the accuracy of the data presented here. However, this data collection exercise was not intended to be used to inform management, purchasing, or clinical decision making, but to test and further develop the measure itself.

Another inadequacy of this trial relates to the fact that many of the patients received their "final score" prior to completion of their treatment, or end of episode of care, to accord with the completion of the research period. Again, this would inadequately reflect the outcomes of some patient groups in these pilot sites, particularly patient groups that are known to progress slowly, that is, learning difficulties/mental retardation.

One of the principles underpinning the development of this approach to outcome measurement is the requirement for a quick, simple way of describing the abilities and deficits of all clients receiving therapy; not just a selected sample of clients. Therefore, it is necessary that the therapist treating the patient should also be the one measuring that patient; any other scenario would be impractical. It is common practice for the treating therapist to also be the assessing therapist, and although this may lead to bias, it can be limited if standardization procedures are adopted and reliability of the measure is robust. However, further work examining the difference between objective and involved raters would be valuable.

DATA COLLECTION FORMS

Data collection forms were designed to assist in experimentation of presentation of the data results (see Appendix D). Some pilot areas required outcome measures to be reported according to medical diagnosis, as this is more appropriate in some directorates and accords with some purchasing directives, whereas others prefer to have the outcomes related to the speech and language diagnosis (see Appendix D1 for coding instructions). Both etiology (medical diagnosis) and impairment (speech and language difficulty) were collected so that the data could be manipulated accordingly.

Each form had a box for personal identification to allow the researchers to contact the individual therapist in the event of inadequate completion. One purpose of the trial was to investigate the practical aspects of using this approach, thus it was necessary to elicit the views and concerns of the users with regard to recording information.

CHAPTER 4

The Outcomes Project Computer System

SYSTEM DESIGN

The hardware platform selected for the development of the system was the standard IBM-compatible personal computer (PC) to commercial specifications; that is, with a 486 processor, at least 4 megabytes of RAM, and a hard disc of >200 megabytes. This specification is met or exceeded by virtually all PCs currently available. The main software was Microsoft Visual Basic. This is a modern development environment that is object-oriented (code is developed in a modular way that facilitates flexibility and reusability) and is capable of controlling and integrating other packages such as databases and spreadsheets. In addition, it has excellent facilities for the design and production of user interfaces such as screen designs. Within the Visual Basic environment, use was made of Microsoft Access Database to store the data, and Microsoft Excel Spreadsheet to analyze the data and to present the reports.

The main aims of the data input module were to minimize errors and ensure that the process was as easy to use as possible. The design strategy was to develop, in parallel, the paper forms on which the data were recorded and the computer screen for data entry. Thus, the structure and appearance were similar in order to minimize transcription errors. Attention was paid at this stage to issues such as whether the data entry clerk would be using the numeric keypad or the main keyboard in order to speed the input of large volumes of data. The software was designed to check and validate each data item as it was entered. This was done using a variety of strategies, including specifying valid numeric ranges and using the features of Visual Basic to allow the data entry clerk to choose only from a list of valid options.

The data are stored in the Microsoft Access Database, a modern relational database system that allows completely flexible retrieval of data items. Although all the data are stored once in a single database file, it was found that useful performance gains, in terms of retrieval time, could be made by creating a range of storage structures that could be applied to the database in the form of indexes.

The generation and presentation of reports was handled by a combination of a Visual Basic interface and Microsoft Excel processing and presentation facilities.

CHAPTER 5

Reliability and Validity Studies

Reliability can be defined as the stability and precision or accuracy of the measure. This is the ability to measure something in a reproducible and consistent fashion (Hammersley, 1987). Assessing the reliability of an adaptation of the outcome measure includes establishing its capacity to replicate results; assessing both interobserver reliability, the degree of agreement between different observers; and assessing the intraobserver reliability, the degree of agreement between observers made by the same judge on two different occasions, demonstrating consistency over time. Any measure will have a degree of error and variability, therefore an acceptable level of reliability of what is considered "good enough" is always required.

Considering the use of the outcome measures, the sample size, and the chances of misclassification, it was judged that the acceptable reliability to be adopted should be 0.8 (Cosby, 1989; Streiner & Norman, 1989). "For purposes of clinical testing reliability coefficients of 0.85 may be considered as indicative of dependable tests" (Rosenthal & Rosnow, 1991). This level would infer a strong relationship and indicate strong similarity of speech and language therapists' scores.

Reliability and validity studies have to be considered carefully. Any measurement that relies on observer inference or self-report is susceptible to halo effects, bias toward leniency or severity, central tendency responses, and position or proximity biases (Bentler & Hamblin, 1986). These factors can artificially enhance the reliability (apparent consistency) of the measurement. A procedure for reducing the influence of measurement bias without losing target specificity is to increase the number of observers, however, the background and expectancies of observers can also exert a contaminating influence (Boroto, Kalafat, & Cohen, 1978). Observer estimates can be made more valid by giving similar training and experience to the raters to help them achieve a criterion level of accuracy. Hence, if differences in measurements are subsequently found, these will be more likely to be attributed to the technique/test rather than the rater (Bentler & Hamblin, 1986).

PILOT RELIABILITY STUDIES

A small pilot project, designed to test the hypothesis that a group of speech and language therapists could be trained to use an adaptation of this measure to an acceptable level of reliability, was conducted principally to test the feasibility of using the approach for a more substantial reliability trial (John, 1993). Some adaptions to the reliability study and the scales themselves were made as the result of this pilot study.

Method

The project involved the adaptation of the outcome measure for children under 6 years of age with language impairment in one district. This was then assessed for the reliability of six participating speech and language therapists who worked within that district.

Results of the Pilot Study

Group 1 rated a video of five children with differing language impairments; these had accompanying composite case histories. The group was shown the tape on two occasions, 2 weeks apart. The inter- and intraobserver ratings were plotted on scattergrams, and a strong positive linear relationship was observed. This allowed the data from the ratings to be analyzed using correlation, while the Spearman Brown formula was used to calculate the effective reliability (Rosenthal & Rosnow, 1991), effective reliability being a measure of the aggregate reliability of the judges, that is, the reliability of the total set of judges, given the number of judges participating.

Table 5–1. Interobserver reliability on TOM pilot study 1.

Domain	1st Rating		2nd Rating	
	Mean	**Effective**	**Mean**	**Effective**
Language Impairment	r.1	R.99	r.91	R.98
Understand/Use Language	r.93	R.98	r.91	R.98
Social Interaction	r.87	R.97	r.85	R.97
Frustration/Upset	r.88	R.97	r.87	R.97

The interobserver reliability of the group is high, with the acceptable level of reliability for the measure achieved in both mean and effective reliability (Table 5–1).

TABLE 5–2. Intraobserver mean and effective reliability on TOM pilot study 1.

Domain	Mean Reliability	Effective Reliability
Language Impairment	r.98	R.99
Understand/Use Language	r.93	R.98
Social Interaction	r.91	R.98
Frustration/Upset	r.92	R.98

Table 5–2 shows the high rate of mean and effective reliability obtained on intraobserver reliability, demonstrating the stability and consistency of the speech and language therapists' judgments using the measure. However, a detailed examination of the speech and language therapists' individual scores and correlations did reveal some patterns of variability. This variability appeared to result from a number of influencing factors such as (a) the ease of rating the particular domains, with the more subjective domains of social interaction and distress demonstrating greater variability than those of impairment and effective understanding/use; (b) difficulties intrinsic to the presenting medium of a video; (c) timing of the training; and (d) train-

ing, with some individuals showing greater variability, which may indicate the requirement for more training for some or that some may be more affected by fatigue.

Subsequent to the first pilot study, some small amendments were made to the adapted outcome measure. This included the addition of .5 to the 0–5 rating scale, as it was anticipated that the additional .5 would add to the scale's precision and accuracy (Nishisato & Torii, 1970; Streiner & Norman, 1989). The adapted outcome measure was then piloted a second time. It was found that given further practice using the measure, with an expanded rate scale, and rating actual cases, a high level of reliability was obtained on each of the Impairment, Disability, Handicap and Wellbeing domains, see Table 5–3.

Table 5–3. Interobserver mean and effective reliability on paired rating of 10 clinical cases of child language disorder.

SLTs	Language Impairment	Disability	Handicap	Wellbeing/ Distress
6 and 1	r .846 R .92	r .906* R .95	r .965*** R .97	r .941* R .95
4 and 5	r .996*** R .99	r .942* R .95	r .976** R .97	r .951** R .95
2 and 3	r .985** R .97	r .987** R .97	r1*** R .99	r1*** R .99

Key: *p > .05, **p > .025, ***p > .01; 1-tailed.

RELIABILITY STUDY

More extensive reliability studies were conducted in four of the eight sites. This larger pilot study had the following specific objectives:

- Does the experience of the speech and language therapists using the outcome measures improve their reliability?
- Do specialized speech and language therapists have greater or lesser reliability when using an outcome measure in their own field of specialization?
- Is reliability affected by whether the therapists have been involved in specific training using the measures?

Procedure

Videos of five patients with dysphasia/aphasia, five patients with learning disability/mental retardation, and five children with language disorders were prepared. The videos of the children and two videos of the patients with dysphasia/aphasia had been made by therapists not involved in this study for general teaching purposes. The other videos were made specifically for this project, but the same material was elicited—the patient was engaged in general conversation and asked some specific questions.[2] The clients were selected to represent a broad range of difficulty, that is, mild to severe impairment. Composite notes were prepared to outline relevant aspects of the case histories.

Two practice cases (videos and notes) were used prior to the reliability study to orientate the participants and discuss details of procedure. Therapists were divided into three groups and the trials were run on three separate days.

Data collection forms allowed identification of the therapist's speciality along with his or her rating of the 15 cases. The results were analyzed using the SPSS package.

Results

Fifty-six therapists rated 15 patients. There was low overall consensus (.68), with greatest agreement on aphasia/dysphasia cases (.72), and worst agreement on learning disability/mental retardation (.62). The variance was not explained by the specialty of the therapist involved. Some therapists included in this reliability study had little or no experience in using the method. These 32 therapists were identified and the data were reanalyzed including only the scores of therapists who had completed 12 or more data collection forms on their own patients.

Experience and practice appear to be critical in reliability. The reanalysis indicated improved overall consensus (.89), with the greatest agreement with the aphasia/dysphasia cases (.92), child language (.88), and the least with learning disability/mental retardation (.84).

The participating therapists found the videos of clients with learning disability/mental retardation difficult to rate as they did not cover a broad range of activities.

Other concerns regarding this trial are:

- The composite notes may have "fed" the score to the therapist.
- The videos were brief and did not reflect issues particularly related to handicap and distress.
- Therapists were unable to interact with a client to confirm or refute an impression.
- Therapists found the task arduous, and concentration waned.

---

[2]Because there was some concern that the video materials chosen may have "primed" the raters, the results of those made by the independent therapists were compared with those made for this project. There was no more or less agreement related to the video.

RELIABILITY STUDY 2

A different approach to calculating reliability was taken in the second study. The four scales are on an 11-point ordinal scale with 0 representing the most severe category and 5 representing normal. Each integer has a corresponding description, and a score of ½ indicates that the subject is slightly better or worse than the description. To assess the interobserver reliability of these scales, the expected agreement by chance needs to be considered. A method that takes into consideration that a disagreement, for example, from 1 to 1½ is not as serious as a disagreement from 1 to 2 is needed. A suitable chance-corrected measure of reliability when there are two observers which takes into consideration the seriousness of different disagreements is the weighted Kappa (Cohen, 1968). The question of what are suitable weights for the weighted Kappa then arises. Streiner and Norman (1989) state that, "unless there are strong prior reasons, the most commonly used weighting scheme, called *quadratic weights*, which bases disagreement weights on the square of the amount of discrepancy, should be used."

By using quadratic weights the weighted Kappa is identical to the intraclass correlation coefficient (Streiner & Norman, 1989) and Maclure and Willett (1987) conclude that, "the weighted Kappa is best when it equals the intraclass correlation coefficient." If the 11 categories in the ordinal scale are assigned discrete values of 1 (most severe) to 11 (normal), quadratic weights in effect quantifies these values.

Reliability coefficients are only summary measures and Landis and Koch (1977) recommended the following interpretations given in Table 5–4.

Table 5–4. Benchmarks for the interpretation of observed Kappa values.

Kappa Statistic	Strength of Agreement
<0.00	Poor
0.00–0.20	Slight
0.21–0.40	Fair
0.41–0.60	Moderate
0.61–0.80	Substantial
0.81–1.00	Almost Perfect

Method

Three separate teams of therapists were involved in rating patients who were presented to them as a group.

Team 1: (Adult team therapists) five therapists rated five patients from different client groups
Team 2: (Community team therapists) nine therapists rated six patients (phonology and child language cases under 5 years)
Team 3: (School team therapists) eight therapists rated five child cases of different types
Team 4: (Whole district team) eight therapists rated eight patients (mixed client group and ages)

Results

The overall group reliability of the teams for the 4 scales are given in Table 5–5.

Table 5–5. The overall group reliability of the teams on the four scales.

Team	Main Impairment	Disability	Handicap	Wellbeing of Subject
Team 1	0.86	0.91	0.46	0.43
Team 2	0.84	0.91	0.91	0.89
Team 3	0.91	0.89	0.74	0.48
Team 4	0.91	0.90	0.64	0.63

Lower reliability of handicap and wellbeing is thought to be the result of insufficient information to allow the therapists to reach consensus.

Conclusion of Reliability Studies

We have collected sufficient information to suggest that this measure has acceptable reliability if the therapist is **trained** and has undertaken a certain **amount of practice**. The specialist skills of the therapist do not seem to affect reliability.

The pilot study and other studies have demonstrated that reliability studies using videos of patient's rather than actual patient's depress reliability scores (Enderby, 1982; John, 1993). Further studies should be undertaken to identify:

■ Interscorer reliability with "live" patients,
■ Exactly how much training and practice is required,
■ Test/retest reliability.

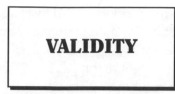

VALIDITY

Face and content validity of this measure can only be assessed through subjective judgment as there is no other measure that could be used for gold standard baseline comparison.

Face validity can be established through:

- expert consensus,
- questionnaires to users that examine validity.

Pilot Validity

Two groups of speech and language therapists involved in the pilot validity trials were required to judge whether the scale appeared appropriate for the intended purposes of measuring child language impairment over four domains.

The expert panels needed to make two judgments concerning the validity of the outcome measure. The following definitions were used (Streiner & Norman, 1989):

1. Face validity: a judgment that the scale looks reasonable; that on the face of it the measure appears to be assessing desired qualities. This represents a subjective judgment based on a review of the measure itself.
2. Content validity: a judgment of whether the measure samples all relevant or important content or domains, that items tap different aspects of the same attribute and not different parts of different traits, and whether the scales were also readable and unambiguous.

There was an introductory talk to reorientate the groups to the Therapy Outcome Measure (TOM), allowing time for discussion of the concepts behind the measures. This included a revision of the original definitions of each of the four domains and an explanation of the process of developing the adapted outcome measure for children with language impairments.

Pilot Results

Face Validity

There was 100% agreement regarding accepting the face validity of the measure. The therapists agreed that the measure appeared to be relevant and sensible and that confidence could be placed in the inferences to be made from the rating of children on such a measure.

Content Validity

The therapists had 100% agreement that the items within each domain tapped different aspects of the same attribute and not different parts or traits. There was less immediate agreement regarding whether the "recognition rules" sampled all relevant or important content or domains. However, there was no consensus on suggestions for inclusions.

VALIDITY STUDY—MAIN STUDY

Forty-seven therapists involved in the main data collection study were sent a brief question-naire. An example of a completed questionnaire can be found in Appendix 5. The results from 35 returned questionnaires showed 100% agreement that using the concepts of impairment, disability, handicap, and wellbeing was relevant to SLTs. A total of 85% (30 therapists) felt that the measures could reflect the changes seen in their patients. However, some of these added qualifying comments such as concern with some client groups (e.g., learning difficulties) and uncertainty regarding reflecting minor changes (i.e., sensitivity). There was general consensus that the domains were appropriate and inclusive.

Analysis of Comments on Forms

At the bottom of each outcome data form therapists were encouraged to write comments to reflect their views/concerns of rating individual patients.

Three hundred comments were received on individual patient's outcome data forms. More than half of these related to explanations of the scores of the individual patient (e.g., "patient did not attend—therefore no change"). Others could be broadly categorized into three areas of concern:

- Concern expressed regarding sensitivity with clients with learning disability/mental retardation.
- Concern regarding the distress/wellbeing score. Therapists were concerned that it was not possible to identify whether it was the patient or the family that was being graded.
- Issues related to grading dual impairments (e.g., cognitive impairment along with language impairment) were raised.

The latter two concerns prompted the changes found in the accompanying user's manual. It is now possible to rate two concurrent impairments. The distress/wellbeing score can now be rated for the client and family separately.

Conclusion of Validity Studies

It is accepted that there is a degree of circularity when the various domains and items were developed from discussions with speech and language therapists to then have therapists rate the face validity, even though they were not the same therapists. However, the feedback allowed some changes to reflect the wishes of a large sample of users. There was demand to allow for measuring dual impairments, as a high proportion of patients have more than one difficulty. General consensus is that wellbeing/distress of families should be monitored separately to that of the client. The published edition of this approach incorporates these changes. Further work on validity needs to be conducted by comparing severity levels from some traditional assessments of speech and language disorders with the impairment level, and traditional assessments of conversation/communication with the disability scale.

CHAPTER 6

Outcome Measure Results

In developing any assessment or measure, it is essential to establish reliability and validity. However, if the measure does not reflect change appropriately or is impractical, the tool will be of little value. This approach was tested on 1,182 patients with results gathered from eight sites (some sites included more than one trust) over a 3-month period; 134 therapists were trained and involved in the data collection.

Details regarding the sites, participants and primary client groups covered are given in Table 6–1.

Table 6–1. Sites, Number of Subjects Included, and Primary Client Groups.

Site	Number of Therapists Involved	Primary Client Groups Covered	Number of Subjects Included
Site 1	20	Fluency disorders, dysphonia, dysphasia/aphasia, dysarthria, dysphagia, developmental language disorders, learning difficulty, phonology, hearing impairment.	148
Site 2	22	Developmental language disorders, phonology, learning disability/mental retardation	335
Site 3	32	Fluency disorders, dysphonia, dysphasia/aphasia, developmental language disorder, learning disability/mental retardation, phonology	232
Site 4	15	Fluency disorders, dysphonia, dysphagia, phonology, developmental language disorders, learning disability/mental retardation	70
Site 5	4	Dysphasia/aphasia	8
Site 6	5	Dysphonia, dysphasia/aphasia, dysphagia, developmental language disorders, learning disability/mental retardation	65
Site 7	20	Fluency disorders, dysphonia, dysphasia/aphasia, dysphagia, learning disability/mental retardation, developmental language disorders, phonology	290
Site 8	14	Fluency disorders, phonology, developmental language disorders, learning disability/mental retardation, dysphagia	34
Total	**132**		**1,182**

Note: At the time subject results were collated for overall results, only 1,171 were available for analysis.

The purpose of this data collection period was to:

- establish whether the measure is sensitive to change;
- establish whether the method could capture and reflect different aspects of change within and between client groups—differential sensitivity;
- establish the acceptability and usability of the approach;
- investigate different ways of collecting and analyzing the data.

CAUTIONS RELATED TO DATA INTERPRETATION

Several caveats must be borne in mind when considering these results:

- This trial was not designed to establish speech and language therapy outcomes for different patient groups, but rather to further standardize the assessment.
- The trial covered, on average, a 3-month period. Many client groups would be expected to show little change over this time period.
- The trial commenced with the summer holidays which affected therapist and client attendance.
- Therapists were asked to recall (using notes) the starting score of an episode of care—this is less likely to be accurate.
- Therapists had to give a "final" score even if episode of care was incomplete.
- Some therapists completed very few outcome scores and did not become familiar with this approach.

The data presented here should not be used to inform service delivery changes.

OVERALL RESULTS

General

Data from 1,182 patients were collected; however, errors and omissions on 11 data forms reduced the number for inclusion. Thus, data from 1,171 patients (from all sites) were collated and analyzed together. See Table (6–2).

Table 6–2. Overall results.

Scoring	I	D	H	W
Starting Score	2.07	2.3	2.25	2.83
Change	0.51	0.64	0.64	0.56
Finishing Score	2.58	2.94	2.89	3.39

Note. In this and the following tables, **I** = Impairment, **D** = Disability, **H** = Handicap, **W** = Wellbeing/Distress. Start is the average score attributed at the beginning of an episode of care. Finish is the average score attributed at the end of an episode of care. Change refers to the difference between start and finish.

As some clients will not (and would not be expected to) change in a particular domain, the number of "no changes" has been identified. However, the percentage change of the average scores is based on the total number. In Table 6–3 it is seen that there is 10.2% overall change in impairment, but 647 of the 1,171 clients did not change in this domain. Thus, the clients that have changed would have changed significantly more than 10%.

Table 6–3. Overall results—identifying number of no changes.

	I		D		H		W	
	Percent Change	Number of No Changes	Percent Change	Number of No Changes	Percent Change	Number of No Changes	Percent Change	Number of No Changes
All patients (1,171)	10.2	647	12.8	523	12.8	541	11.2	647

Two hundred and fifty-six clients did not change or showed a negative change on all domains. Two hundred and thirty-six patients changed on one domain and 678 patients changed on two or more domains.

Etiology

The term *etiology* was used to ascribe a medical diagnosis to the patient. Of the 1,171 subjects, the largest subgroups were as follows:

- Developmental delay (learning disability/mental retardation)   288
- Nothing abnormal detected; no medical diagnosis[3]   161
- Acquired neurological disease   158
- Syndromes   138
- Multifactorial (mostly elderly)   146
- Voice pathology   76

Results related to etiology indicate that the greatest change in impairment can be seen in voice pathology (1.59) and cardiovascular disease (1.04). The greatest changes in disability can be seen in cardiovascular disease (1.66), voice pathology (1.36), and acquired neurological (1.16). The greatest changes in handicap can be seen in cardiovascular disease (1.87), voice pathology (1.49), orofacial/neck surgery (1.33), and acquired neurological (1.15). The greatest change in wellbeing can be seen in cardiovascular disease (1.75), voice pathology (1.66), and neurosurgery (1.0) (see Table 6–4).

The impairment score for "progressive neurological disease" was the only domain showing deterioration. Little or no change is seen in the client groups burns/plastics (1 patient only), and cerebral palsy (41 patients).

---

[3] These would be predominantly clients with delayed development of speech or language or those with disorders of fluency.

Table 6–4. Overall outcome scores by etiologies.

Etiology (No. of Patients)	I	D	H	W
Cardiovascular Disease (24)				
Start	1.89	2.12	1.7	2.41
Change	1.04	1.66	1.87	1.75
Finish	2.93	3.78	3.57	4.16
Acquired Neurological (158)				
Start	2.32	1.95	1.77	2.65
Change	0.96	1.16	1.15	0.8
Finish	3.28	3.11	2.92	3.45
Neurosurgery (2)				
Start	2.5	2.5	2.5	2.5
Change	1.0	1.5	1.0	1.0
Finish	3.5	4.0	3.5	3.5
Orofacial/Neck Surgery (6)				
Start	2.33	2.5	2.0	2.83
Change	1.0	0.91	1.33	0.91
Finish	3.33	3.41	3.33	3.74
Progressive Neurological Disease (14)				
Start	1.67	2.42	3.0	2.96
Change	-0.03	0.75	0.14	0.07
Finish	1.64	3.17	3.14	3.03
Voice Pathology (76)				
Start	2.3	2.51	2.64	2.28
Change	1.59	1.36	1.49	1.66
Finish	3.89	3.87	4.13	3.94
Burns/Plastic (1)				
Start	3.0	3.0	3.0	4.0
Change	0.0	0.5	0.0	0.0
Finish	3.0	3.5	3.0	4.0
Development Delay (288)				
Start	2.18	2.44	2.41	3.07
Change	0.48	0.56	0.56	0.37
Finish	2.66	3.00	2.97	3.44
Cerebral Palsy (41)				
Start	1.68	2.03	1.96	3.2
Change	0.04	0.15	0.24	0.12
Finish	1.72	2.18	2.2	3.32
Multifactorial (140)				
Start	1.63	1.91	1.76	2.71
Change	0.17	0.29	0.36	0.27
Finish	1.80	2.20	2.12	2.98

Nothing Abnormal Detected (161)				
Start	2.38	2.56	2.76	2.92
Change	0.69	0.79	0.69	0.78
Finish	3.07	3.35	3.45	3.70
Syndromes(138)				
Start	2.01	2.28	2.25	3.11
Change	0.16	0.3	0.23	0.19
Finish	2.17	2.58	2.48	3.30
Others(122)				
Start	2.06	2.38	2.09	2.49
Change	0.09	0.38	0.39	0.36
Finish	2.15	2.76	2.48	2.85

Table 6–5 indicates that a high percentage of some client groups did not change on impairment; for example, 145/288 with developmental delay, 12/14 progressive neurological disease, 36/41 cerebral palsy, and 103/135 multifactorial. However, the majority of clients in the groups, voice pathology, NAD, and acquired neurological conditions showed some gain in this domain. Overall, more clients in all the client groups showed change in the areas of disability (504/1,171 no changes) and handicap (529/1,171 no changes).

Table 6–5. Overall outcomes etiologies-numbers of no changes.

Etiologiccs	% Change in I	Number of No Change	% Change in D	Number of No Change	% Change in H	Number of No Change	% Change in W	Number of No Change
Cardiovascular Disease (24)	20.8	7	33.2	1	37.4	2	35	6
Acquired Neurological (158)	19.2	49	23.2	43	23	51	16	64
Neurosurgery (2)	20	0	30	0	20	0	20	1
Orofacial/Neck Surgery (6)	20	3	18.2	2	18.2	1	26.6	1
Progressive Neurological Disease (14)	–0.6	12	15	5	2.8	12	1.4	12
Voice Pathology (76)	31.8	12	27.2	14	29.8	15	33.2	8
Burns/Plastics (1)	0	1	10	0	0	1	0	1
Developmental Delay (288)	9.6	145	11.2	137	11.2	136	7.4	180
Cerebral Palsy (41)	0.8	36	3	30	4.8	25	2.4	32
Multifactorial (135)	3.4	103	5.8	82	7.2	75	5.4	95
Nothing Abnormal Detected (161)	13.8	60	15.8	50	13.8	60	15.6	72
Syndromes (138)	3.2	103	6	75	4.6	85	3.8	99
Others (122)	1.8	100	7.6	65	7.8	66	7.2	65

Impairment

The same underlying medical diagnosis may give rise to different speech/language disorders; and conversely, a particular speech/language disorder could be caused by different underlying medical/psychological pathology. Therefore, it is possible that the outcome results would indicate different trends if the results were clustered according to the speech and language diagnosis. Fifteen speech and language diagnoses were identified. However, no laryngectomy patients were included in this trial. Some other patients with more obscure difficulties were clustered in a category called "other." Thus, data are available on 14 specific speech and language categories and "other."

Inspection of Table 6–6 shows that the largest gains in all domains can be seen in:

- Disorders of voice
- Dysphagia
- Dysphasia/Aphasia
- Developmental language disorders
- Phonological disorders.

Small gains overall were seen in:

- Learning disability
- Autism
- Dyspraxia.

It is interesting to note that dysarthria (18 patients) shows little gain on impairment (3.8%) but worthwhile gains in disability (15%), handicap (12.2%), and wellbeing (15.4%). Similarly, disorders of fluency (stammering, 41 patients) show less gain on impairment (9.6%) but greater gains in disability (16%), handicap (19.6%), and wellbeing (25.2%).

The sensitivity of the test to change was established by using a t Test which demonstrated varying degrees of change related to the impairment (See Table 6–7).

Table 6–6. Overall outcomes impairments including numbers of no changes.

	% Change in I	Number of No Change	% Change in D	Number of No Change	% Change in H	Number of No Change	% Change in W	Number of No Change
Disorders of Fluency (41)	9.6	21	16	13	19.6	13	25.2	11
Disorders of Voice (79)	30.8	14	26.4	16	28	20	32	11
Laryngectomy (0)	NO PATIENTS							
Acquired Language Disorder (95) (Dysphasia)	16.4	31	20.8	21	23.2	28	15.4	40
Dyslexia (4)	5	2	0	4	7.4	3	22.4	1
Acquired Speech Disorder (18) (Dysarthria)	3.8	11	15	7	12.2	9	15	11
Dyspraxia (15)	9.2	7	14.6	4	8.6	7	10	6
Dysphagia (69)	25.2	23	32	20	28.2	26	24.2	26
Autism (25)	4.4	17	10	11	7.2	14	7.2	14
Developmental Disorder of Language (183)	13.8	72	16.2	59	14.4	64	12.2	86
Articulation Impairment (6)	6.6	4	3.2	5	11.6	3	13.2	4
Phonological Impairment (161)	12.4	55	10.8	72	10.6	81	6.8	98
Deaf Speech/Language (13)	4.6	9	6	8	15.2	4	15.2	5
Cleft Palate Speech (5)	14	2	12	3	12	3	14	3
Learning Disability (457)	1.8	368	5.2	273	5.8	256	4	320
Others (14)	5.6	10	7	7	3.4	9	8.4	9

Table 6–7. Overall outcomes by speech/language impairments.

Impairment (No. of Clients)	I	D	H	W	t=test
Disorder of Fluency (41)					
Start	2.73	2.74	2.59	2.34	.0062
Change	0.48	0.8	0.98	1.26	
Finish	3.21	3.55	3.58	3.6	
Disorder of Voice (79)					
Start	2.35	2.57	2.71	2.34	.0000
Change	1.54	1.32	1.4	1.6	
Finish	3.89	3.89	4.12	3.94	
Acquired Language Disorder (95) (Dysphasia/Aphasia)					
Start	1.82	1.89	1.75	2.78	.0010
Change	0.82	1.04	1.16	0.77	
Finish	2.64	2.93	2.92	3.56	
Dyslexia (4)					
Start	2.0	4.5	3.0	2.5	.0844
Change	0.25	0.0	0.37	1.12	
Finish	2.25	4.5	3.37	3.62	
Acquired Speech Disorders (18) Dysarthria					
Start	2.08	2.88	3.27	2.91	.0113
Change	0.19	0.75	0.61	0.75	
Finish	2.27	3.63	3.88	3.66	
Dyspraxia (15)					
Start	1.56	2.03	2.09	2.6	.0020
Change	0.46	0.73	0.43	0.5	
Finish	2.03	2.76	2.53	3.1	
Dysphagia (69)					
Start	2.18	2.05	1.76	2.4	.0003
Change	1.26	1.6	1.41	1.21	
Finish	3.44	3.65	3.18	3.62	
Autism (25)					
Start	1.0	1.42	1.2	1.5	.0040
Change	0.22	0.5	0.36	0.36	
Finish	1.22	1.92	1.56	1.86	
Developmental Disorder of Language (183)					
Start	2.02	2.1	2.17	2.71	.0002
Change	0.69	0.81	0.72	0.61	
Finish	2.72	2.91	2.89	3.32	

(continued)

Table 6–7. *(continued)*

Impairment (No. of Clients)	I	D	H	W	t=test
Articulation Impairment (6)					
Start	2.83	3.5	3.16	3.5	.0165
Change	0.33	0.16	0.58	0.66	
Finish	3.16	3.66	3.75	4.16	
Phonological Impairment (161)					
Start	2.78	3.02	3.18	3.68	.0017
Change	0.62	0.54	0.53	0.34	
Finish	3.4	3.57	3.72	4.02	
Deaf Speech/Language (13)					
Start	1.46	1.92	1.69	2.0	.0184
Change	0.23	0.3	0.76	0.76	
Finish	1.69	2.23	2.46	2.76	
Cleft Plate (5)					
Start	2.0	2.6	2.8	2.6	.0000
Change	0.7	0.6	0.6	0.7	
Finish	2.7	3.2	3.4	3.3	
Learning Disability/Mental Retardation (457)					
Start	1.84	2.17	2.03	2.88	.0092
Change	0.09	0.26	0.29	0.2	
Finish	1.93	2.44	2.33	3.09	
Others (14)					
Start	2.71	3.0	2.6	3.32	.0048
Change	0.28	0.35	0.17	0.42	
Finish	3.0	3.35	2.78	3.75	

Contacts

The number of contacts related to an episode of care was collected to test the analysis of relating change to contacts. Table 6–8 demonstrates this but also shows that doing a composite analysis is uninformative. Later in this report the change/contacts of a specific client group allows access to more meaningful and identifiable information.

Results by Age

Analyzing outcome of all 1,171 patients by age, disregarding etiology or impairment, is again generally uninformative. However, some general impressions can be gained. It appears that influencing change in the age range of 11–19 years is particularly difficult (but most of these clients are likely to be learning disabled/mentally retarded). Influencing all domains in the age

Table 6–8. Overall outcomes by contacts.

Number of Contacts	I	D	H	W
1 Only (22)				
Start	2.76	2.76	2.93	3.32
Change	0.56	0.78	0.8	0.82
Finish	3.32	3.54	3.73	4.15
2 TO 5 (292)				
Start	2.35	2.43	2.5	2.95
Change	0.53	0.65	0.55	0.54
Finish	2.89	3.09	3.05	3.49
6 TO 10 (387)				
Start	2.18	2.47	2.39	2.93
Change	0.52	0.63	0.69	0.56
Finish	2.7	3.1	3.08	3.5
11 TO 20 (284)				
Start	1.84	2.15	2.02	2.78
Change	0.42	0.57	0.62	0.53
Finish	2.26	2.72	2.65	3.31
21 TO 30 (77)				
Start	1.71	1.92	1.84	2.44
Change	0.5	0.69	0.61	0.5
Finish	2.22	2.62	2.46	2.94
31 TO 50 (72)				
Start	1.6	1.92	1.91	2.27
Change	0.72	0.82	0.7	0.72
Finish	2.32	2.75	2.62	3
51 TO 70 (20)				
Start	1.6	2.07	1.67	2.7
Change	0.72	0.8	0.7	0.4
Finish	2.32	2.87	2.37	3.1
71 TO 100 (6)				
Start	1.25	1.5	0.83	2.16
Change	1.16	1.25	2	1.41
Finish	2.41	2.75	2.83	3.58
100 + (1)				
Start	2	3	2	3
Change	–2	–1	–1	0
Finish	0	2	1	3

range of 61 years and older appears to be more effective (but most patients in this group are likely to have acute difficulties). Later analysis of relating age to both etiology and impairment again accesses more useful information (see Table 6–9).

Table 6–9. Overall outcomes by age ranges.

Age Range	I	D	H	W
0 TO 3 (134)				
Start	2.05	1.99	2.19	2.55
Change	0.67	0.85	0.74	0.76
Finish	2.72	2.84	2.94	3.32
4 TO 5 (206)				
Start	2.23	2.49	2.59	3.33
Change	0.61	0.59	0.54	0.38
Finish	2.84	3.08	3.13	3.72
6 TO 10 (181)				
Start	2.01	2.44	2.36	3.09
Change	0.41	0.52	0.5	0.33
Finish	2.43	2.97	2.87	3.43
11 TO 19 (57)				
Start	2.3	2.45	2.42	2.92
Change	0.05	0.17	0.27	0.21
Finish	2.35	2.62	2.69	3.14
20 TO 40 (235)				
Start	2.08	2.39	2.18	2.65
Change	0.18	0.4	0.43	0.41
Finish	0.59	2.8	2.62	3.06
41 TO 60 (160)				
Start	1.88	2.23	2.09	2.58
Change	0.59	0.65	0.72	0.7
Finish	2.48	2.89	2.81	3.28
61 + (103)				
Start	2.03	2.1	1.99	2.62
Change	0.91	1.12	1.16	1.01
Finish	2.95	3.23	3.15	3.63

Results by Site

The detailed results of each participating site are available in Appendixes F–M. Although this trial was not designed to evaluate the effectiveness of therapy, but rather to test sensitivity, differential sensitivity, and practicality of the measures, it is of interest to demonstrate the value of having a unified approach to describing outcome which allows for comparisons in outcomes between sites. This is illustrated by examining the results in different sites. Table 6–10 details the outcome scores of dysphasic/aphasic clients treated in five sites.

Proportionally, Site 7 had the most patients resistant to change in each domain and less overall gain (see Table 6–10). There was also a decrease in the wellbeing score which contra-

Table 6–10. Comparison of outcome scores for clients with dysphasia/aphasia in five sites.

Site	No. of Subjects	Impairment			Disability			Handicap			Wellbeing		
		Start	Change	Finish	Start	Change	Finish	Start	Change	Finish	Start	Change	Finish
Site 5	(8)	2	1.12 (22.4%) 2 No change	3.12	1.87	1.25 (25%) 1 No change	3.12	1.87	1.5 (30%) 3 No change	3.37	3	1.12 (22.4%) 1 No change	4.12
Site 1	(17)	2.23	1.08 (21.6%) 4 No change	3.31	2.35	1.41 (28.2%) 3 No change	3.76	2.61	1.61 (32.2%) 4 No change	4.22	2.76	1.55 (31%) 6 No change	4.31
Site 7	(11)	1.72	0.36 (7.2%) 5 No change	2.08	2	0.63 (12.6%) 3 No change	2.63	1.72	0.72 (14.4%) 6 No change	2.44	2.9	−0.13 (−2.6%) 7 No change	2.77
Site 6	(20)	2.27	0.61 (12.2%) 5 No change	2.88	2.25	0.52 (10.4%) 8 No change	2.77	1.27	1.05 (21%) 4 No change	2.33	1.91	0.63 (12.6%) 8 No change	2.54
Site 3	(34)	1.47	0.58 (11.6%) 16 No change	2.05	1.61	1.07 (21.4%) 6 No change	2.68	1.66	0.95 (19%) 10 No change	2.61	3.04	0.36 (7.2%) 17 No change	3.40

dicts the trend of the other sites. This ocurred despite the fact that their patients are not particularly different from those at other sites at baseline.

Table 6–11 compares outcome data of each of four sites with fluency disorders. Site 1 appears to have a cohort of patients with less difficulties than the other sites. Site 3 appears to influence positively a higher number of patients to a greater extent and the clients in site 8 show less change overall.

Table 6–12 compares the results of children with phonological problems treated in five sites. None show striking changes in wellbeing which may not be a component of therapy effort for this client group. Site 4 has a higher percentage of "no changes" for impairment; however, there are some similarities in outcomes. Noticeably higher gains in the domains of handicap and impairment are achieved by site 3 as compared to the other sites, whereas site 8 appears to have a less favorable impact overall.

These comparisons stimulate many questions, for example:

- Why do the initial scores of some client groups' seem markedly different?
- Is this related to referral policy?
- Why do some client groups in some sites seem more resistant to change?
- Is this related to severity of condition, type of intensity or therapy?

A study specifically designed to compare outcomes in different sites would need methodology to ensure that similar patient groups were compared (by matching age, specific aspects of etiology, etc.) and the data were collected over the complete course of treatment (beginning to end). This was not done in this study. These data illustrate that outcome measures may assist in aspects of care that warrant further investigation.

Table 6–11. Comparison of outcome scores in four sites for fluency disorders.

Site	No. of Subjects	Impairment			Disability			Handicap			Wellbeing		
		Start	Change	Finish	Start	Change	Finish	Start	Change	Finish	Start	Change	Finish
Site 1	(8)	3.75	0.06 (1.2%) 2 No change	3.81	3.56	0.37 (7.4%) 1 No change	3.93	3	1 (20%) 2 No change	4	2.75	1.43 (28.6%) 2 No change	4.18
Site 3	(7)	2.14	1.14 (22.8%) 3 No change	3.28	1.92	1.42 (28.4%) 2 No change	3.34	1.92	1.5 (30%) 1 No change	3.42	1.85	1.71 (34.2%) 2 No change	3.56
Site 4	(5)	2.8	0.8 (16%) 2 No change	3.6	2.4	2 (40%) 0 No change	4.4	2.6	2 (40%) 0 No change	4.6	2.4	2 (40%) 0 No change	4.4
Site 8	(9)	2.55	–0.16 (–3.2%) 7 No change	2.39	2.55	0.33 (6.6%) 5 No change	2.88	2.66	0.27 (5.4%) 4 No change	2.93	2.55	0.5 (10%) 3 No change	3.05

Table 6–12. Comparison of outcome scores in five sites for phonology.

Site	No. of Subjects	Impairment			Disability			Handicap			Wellbeing		
		Start	Change	Finish	Start	Change	Finish	Start	Change	Finish	Start	Change	Finish
Site 1	(31)	3.22	0.58 (11.6%) 4 No change	3.8	2.9	0.82 (16.4%) 4 No change	3.72	3.58	0.37 (7.4%) 1 No change	3.95	4.01	0.22 (4.4%) 2 No change	4.23
Site 3	(42)	2.58	0.88 (21.6%) 4 No change	3.46	3.0	0.63 (12.6%) 20 No change	3.63	2.86	0.77 (15.4%) 20 No change	3.63	3.57	0.43 (9%) 24 No change	4
Site 4	(13)	2.5	0.8 (16%) 7 No change	3.3	3.38	0.5 (10%) 9 No change	3.88	4.19	0.3 (6%) 12 No change	4.49	4.13	0.38 (7.6%) 10 No change	4.51
Site 7	(56)	2.72	0.54 (10.8%) 23 No change	3.26	3.02	0.41 (8.2%) 30 No change	3.43	3.03	0.5 (10%) 30 No change	3.53	3.45	0.36 (7.2%) 39 No change	3.81
Site 8	(34)	3.0	0.33 (6.6%) 5 No change	3.33	3.22	0.33 (6.6%) 5 No change	3.55	3.11	0.44 (8.8%) 4 No change	3.55	4	0 (0%) 7 No change	4

CHAPTER 7

Conclusion

This study was challenging as it involved more than 100 therapists in eight geographical sites and produced more than 1,000 patient results.

The philosophy of the WHO classification lends itself well to speech and language therapy and other rehabilitation professions. The WHO terminology allows the diversity of the difficulties experienced by patients to be reflected and the different emphasis of therapy to be displayed. Different client groups require different therapeutic targets: Some groups will need more traditional "medical" involvement to remedy the impairment, whereas others may benefit from an emphasis on social/counseling. Therapists must be able to expose the features of treatment, not only to review their effectiveness with individual and groups of clients, but also to demonstrate the services provided so that purchasers can more fully appreciate that speech and language therapy is more than "getting people to talk." The different scales developed by the participating sites have been amalgamated to form composite scales that are available in the accompanying user's manual.

Many philosophical difficulties remain in the field of outcome measurement, one of the most fundamental being the near impossibility of relating an input to an outcome in a clinical situation. For example, improved speech/language or coping strategies in an individual client may be due to good multidisciplinary teamwork or environmental changes, rather than the speech and language therapist's efforts per se. However, being able to describe groups of patients more accurately should inform discussion and allow change to be monitored, assisting attribution to be examined.

Austin and Clark, (1993) focused attention on the different perspectives held by clinician, patients, caregivers, and managers regarding the same outcome. They expressed concerns related to the insight of patients and caregivers, individuality of patient expectations, frequency of co-morbidity, and conflicting goals. It is therefore essential to remember that outcome measures produce data and not information. It is only when the data are put in to context, considered, and interpreted that we will become better informed.

This study has developed an approach to outcome measurement which grew out of an analysis of what therapy aims to achieve. The approach has proved reliable (when therapists are given basic training and allowed some practice), valid, sensitive to change, and may allow comparison of services. However, considerable further work is required, not only in standardizing and developing the approach, but also in using this approach in evaluation of speech and language therapy. Furthermore, outcome measurement, as viewed by patients and caregivers, is likely to teach us a great deal and assist in improving tailoring services to meet user needs (see Appendix N).

"How many of you get desirable outcomes? (Most raise their hands). How do you know? (Most quickly lower their hands). Because you are certified, licensed and come from an accredited program? Not good enough. We want efficacy data. We want outcome data. We want cost/benefit data. We are the policymakers, payers, clients. We are your consumers. And you exist because you say you can meet our needs. Prove it! There is no substitute for knowledge."

—C. Frattali (September 1991, p. 12)

REFERENCES

Anderson, J., Sullivan, F., & Usherwood, T. (1990). The Medical Outcomes Study Instrument (MOST): Use of a new health status measure in Britain. *Family Practice, 7*, 205–218.

Andrews, F., & Crandal, R. (1976). The validity of measures of self reported wellbeing. *Social Indicators Research, 3*, 1–19.

Austin, C., & Clark, C. R. (1993). Measures of outcome: For whom?. *British Journal of Occupational Therapy, 56*, 21–24.

Bentler, L. E., & Hamblin, D. L. (1986). Individualized outcome measures of internal change: Methodological considerations. *Journal of Consulting and Clinical Psychology, 54*, 46–53.

Bishop, D. V. M., & Edmundson, A. (1987). Specific language impairment as a maturational lag: Evidence from longitudinal data on language and motor development. *Developmental Medicine and Child Neurology, 19*, 442–449.

Blomert, L. (1990). What functional assessment can contribute to setting goals for aphasia therapy. *Aphasiology, 4*, 307–320.

Boroto, D. R., Kalafat, J.D., & Cohen, L. H. (1978). Clients vs rater judgments of counsellor effectiveness. *Journal of Clinical Psychology, 34*, 188–194.

Byers-Brown, B., & Edwards, M. (1989). *Developmental disorders of language.* London: Whurr.

Cantwell, D. P., & Baker, L. (1987). Prevalence and type of psychiatric disorders in three speech and language groups. *Journal of Communication Disorders, 20*, 151–160.

Cochrane, A. L. (1972). *Effectiveness and efficiency: Random reflections on health services.* London: Nuffield Provincial Hospital Trust.

Cohen, J. (1968). Weighted Kappa: Nominal scale agreement with provision for scaled disagreement or partial credit. *Psychological Bulletin, 70*, 213–220.

Cosby, J. (1989). *Methods in behavioral research.* Los Angeles, CA: Mayfield.

Cowley, A. J., Fullwood, L. J., Muller, A. F., Stainer, K., Skene, A. M., & Hampton, J. R. (1991). Exercise capability in heart failure: Is cardiac output important after all. *Lancet, 33*, 771–773.

Crowley, C. (1992). Behavioral difficulties and their relationships to language impairment. In J. Law (Ed.), *The early identification of language impairment in children* (pp. 63–84). London: Chapman & Hall.

Department of Health. (1989). Working for patients. *Working Papers*, 1–6. London: HMSO.

Department of Health. (1993). *Improving clinical effectiveness.* Executive Letter: EL (93) 115.

Donaldson, S. W., Vagner, C. C., & Gresham, G. E. (1973). A unified ADL evaluation form. *Archives of Physical Medicine and Rehabilitation, 54*, 175–179.

Donovan, J. L., Frankel, S. J., & Eyles, J. D. (1993). Assessing the need for health status measures. *Journal of Epidemiology and Community Health, 47*, 158–162.

Ebrahim, S., Nouri, F., & Barer, D. (1985). Measuring disability after a stroke. *Journal of Epidemiology Community Health, 39*, 86–89.

Enderby, P. (1981). Frenchay Dysarthria Assessment. *British Journal of Disorders of Communication, 15*, 165–173.

Enderby, P. (1982). *The assessment of dysarthria.* Doctoral dissertation, Bristol Medical School.

Enderby, P. (1992). Outcome measures in speech therapy: Impairment, disability, handicap and distress. *Health Trends, 24*, 61–64.

Frattali, C. (1991, September). Professional practices perspective. *Asha, 33*, 12.

Fugl-Meyer, A. R., Branholm, I. B., & Fugl-Meyer, K. S. (1991). Happiness and domain specific life satisfaction in adult northern Swedes. *Clinical Rehabilitation, 5*, 25–33.

Goldberg, D., & Hillier, V. (1979). A scaled version of the general health questionnaire. *Psychological Medicine, 9*, 139–145.

Haley, S. M., Coster, W. J., & Ludlow, L. H. (1991). Pediatric functional outcome measures. *Physical Medicine and Rehabilitation Clinics of North America, 2*, 689–723.

Hammersley, M. (1987). Some notes on the terms "validity" and "reliability". *British Educational Research Journal, 13*, 73–81.

Harewood, R. H., Jitapunkel, S., Dickenson, E., & Ebrahim, S. (1994). Measuring handicap: Motives, methods and a model. *Quality in Health Care, 3*, 53–57.

Health Care Advisory Board. (1994). Quality measures: Next generation of outcome tracking. *The Advisory Board, 2*, 25, 32.

Hopkins, A. (1993, Spring). Why measure outcome? *Outcome Briefing*, pp. 16–20.

Hunt, S., & McEwen, J. (1980). The development of a subjective health indicator. *Social Health and Illness, 2*, 231–246.

John, A. K. M. (1993). *An outcome measure for language impaired children under 6 years: A study of reliability and validity.* Master's thesis, City University.

Langton Hewer, R. (1990). Outcome measures in stroke. A British view. *Stroke, 21*(Suppl. II) 11–55.

Maclure, M., & Willett, W. C. (1987). Misinterpretation and misuse of the Kappa statistic. *American Journal of Epidemiology, 126,* 161–169.

McCrae, R. R., & Costa, P. T. (1986). Personality, coping and coping effectiveness in an adult sample. *Journal of Personality, 2,* 285–405.

McKenna, S. P., Hunt, S. M., & Tennant, A. (1993). The development of a patient completed index of distress from the Nottingham Health Profile: A new measure for use in cost utility studies. *British Journal of Medical Economics, 6,* 13–24.

Meenan, R., Gertman, P., & Mason, J. (1980). Measuring health status in arthritis. *Arthritis and Rheumatism, 23,* 146–152.

Melzack, R. (Ed.). (1983). *Pain measurement and assessment.* New York: Raven Press.

Nishisato, N., & Torii, Y. (1970). Effects on categorizing normal distributions on the product-moment correlation. *Japanese Psychological Research, 13,* 45–49.

Patrick, D., Darby, S., Green, S., Horton, G., Locker, D., & Wiggins, R. (1981). Screening for disability in the inner city. *Journal of Epidemiology and Community Health, 35,* 65–70.

Riesenberg, D., & Glass, R. M. (1989). The medical outcomes study. *JAMA, 262,* 943.

Rosenthal, R., & Rosnow, R. L. (1991). *Essentials of behavioral research methods of data analysis.* Series in Psychology (2nd ed., p. 82). New York: McGraw Hill.

Rosser, R. M. (1976). Recent studies using a global approach to measuring illness. *Medical Care, 14*(Suppl. 5), 138–147.

Royal College of Speech and Language Therapists. (1996). *Communication quality.* London.

Sarno, M. T. (1993). Aphasia rehabilitation psychosocial and ethical considerations. *Aphasiology, 7,* 321–334.

Scott, J., & Huskisson, E. C. (1979). Vertical or horizontal visual analogue scales. *Annals of Rheumatic Disorders, 38,* 560.

Spitzer, W. O., Dobson, A. J., & Hall, J. (1981). Measuring quality of life of cancer patients: A concise QL-Index for use by physicians. *Journal of Chronic Disorders, 34,* 585–597.

Stephen, D., & Hetu, R. (1992). Impairment, disability and handicap in audiology: Towards a consensus. *Audiology,* 1–15.

Stewart, A. L., Greenfield, S., Hays, R., Wells, K., Rogers, W., Berry, S., McGlynn, E., & Ware, J. (1989). Functional status and wellbeing of patients with chronic conditions: Results from a medical outcome study. *JAMA, 262,* 909–913.

Streiner, D. L., & Norman, G. R. (1989). *Health measurement scales:* A practical guide to their development and use (Chap. 8). New York: Oxford University Press.

Wade, D. (1992). *Measurement in neurological rehabilitation.* Oxford: Oxford University Press.

Ware, J. E. (1991). Conceptualising and measuring generic health outcomes. *Cancer, 67*(Suppl.), 774–779.

Wertz, R. T. (1983). A philosophy of aphasia therapy. Some things patients do not say but that you can see if you listen. *Communication Disorders, 8,* 1–17.

Wertz, R. T. (1987). Language therapy for aphasics is efficacious, but for whom? *Topics of Language Disorders, 8,* 1–10.

Wertz, R. T. (1993, January). Issues in treatment efficacy: Adult onset disorders. We would like to know how much works best for whom. *Asha, 35,* 38–39.

Whiteneck, S., Charlifue, S. W., Gerhart, K. A., Overholson, J. D., & Richardson, N. (1992). Quantifying handicap: A new measure of long-term rehabilitation outcomes. *Archives of Physical and Medical Rehabilitation, 73,* 519–525.

Wilkin, D., Hallam, L., & Doggett, M. (1992). *Measures of need and outcome for primary health care.* Oxford: Oxford University Press.

Williams, A., Ware, J., & Donald, C. (1981). A model of mental health, life events and social supports applicable to general populations. *Journal of Health and Social Behavior, 22,* 324–336.

Williams, S. J., & Bury, M. R. (1989). "Breathtaking" the consequence of chronic respiratory disorder. *International Disability Studies, 11,* 114–120.

Wood, P. H. N., & Badley, E. M. (1978). An epidemiological appraisal of disablement. In A. E. Bennett (Ed.), *Recent advances in community medicine.* Edinburgh: Churchill Livingstone.

Wood, P. H. (1980). The language of disablement: A glossary relating to disease and its consequences. *International Rehabilitation Medicine, 2,* 86–92.

APPENDIX A

Pilot Core Scale

Impairment

0   The most severe presentation of this impairment.
1   Severe presentation of this impairment.
2   Severe/moderate presentation.
3   Moderate presentation.
4   Just below normal/mild presentation.
5   No impairment.

Disability

0   Totally dependent/unable to function.
1   Assists/cooperates but burden of task/achievement falls on professional or caregiver.
2   Can undertake some part of task but needs a high level of support to complete.
3   Can undertake task/function in familiar situation but requires some verbal/physical assistance.
4   Requires some minor assistance occasionally or extra time to complete task.
5   Independent/able to function.

Handicap

0   No autonomy, isolated, no social/family role.
1   Very limited choices, contact mainly with professionals, no social or family role, little control over life.
2   Some integration, value, and autonomy in one setting.
3   Integrated, valued, and autonomous in limited number of settings.
4   Occasionally some restriction in autonomy, integration, or role.
5   Integrated, valued, occupies appropriate role.

APPENDIX B

Examples of Scales for Dysphasia/Aphasia Produced by Four Different Sites

APHASIA (INCLUDING DYSPRAXIC OUTPUT)

Impairment

Rate each on R = Reception, E = Expression

0   Global dysphasia/aphasia can include total apraxia (severe)
    R: No understanding of words
    E: No accurate vocabulary
1   Small amount of accurate vocabulary understood or expressed occasionally (severe/ moderate)
2   Limited understanding of accurate vocabulary understood or expressed occasionally (severe/moderate)
3   Can understand and express moderately well (mild/moderate)
4   Mild expressive or receptive difficulty occasionally apparent (mild)
5   Normal

Disability/Functional Communication

0   No effective communication
1   Minimal communication with maximal assistance
2   Able to communicate basic needs but listener assists significantly
3   Able to communicate more widely with less listener support but with a degree of inconsistency
4   Can communicate effectively without assistance but may be limited by the situation
5   Converse at premorbid level

Handicap/Social Interaction

0   A feeling of isolation and lack of control
1   Severely limited confidence with little control
2   Lacks confidence in the majority of settings
3   Confident in a limited number of settings
4   Only occasional difficulties with confidence
5   Confident

Wellbeing/Distress

0   Severe constant distress
1   Frequent severe distress
2   Moderate constant distress
3   Frequent mild or moderate distress
4   Occasional mild or moderate distress
5   No distress

DYSPHASIA/APHASIA

Impairment

0   Severe dysphasia/aphasia.
1   Severe dysphasia/aphasia but small amount of vocabulary used occasionally.
2   Speech effortful/small vocabulary that can be used appropriately and purposefully.
3   Can understand and express moderately well with effort.
4   Mild expressive or receptive difficulties occasionally apparent.
5   No language defect.

Disability (Communicative Effectiveness)

0   Unable to communicate in any way.
1   Can communicate very occasionally.
2   Can understand and make self understood to family members only.
3   Can make self understood and can understand consistently but at a moderate level.
4   Occasionally has difficulty understanding or getting message across. Some difficulty in some situations.
5   Communicates well in all situations.

Handicap (Associated Consequence)

0   Isolated/no control over life.
1   Lacks confidence. Low self-esteem.
2   Has control over only a limited number of aspects. Feels some confidence in restricted settings.
3   Relates well in environment. Confidence is easily broken. Diffident about general control over life.
4   Occasionally has difficulties with self-confidence and self-esteem.
5   Is involved in controlling life. Feels appropriately valued and confident.

Wellbeing/Distress

0   Very embarrassed/frustrated and upset all the time.
1   Frequent severely embarrassed/upset/frustrated.
2   Feels moderately embarrassed, upset or frustrated most of the time.
3   Frequent periods of embarrassment, upset, or frustration.
4   Occasional periods of mild upset, distress, or embarrassment.
5   No inappropriate distress, upset, or embarrassment.

DYSPHASIA/APHASIA

Impairment

0 Severe dysphasia/aphasia in all modalities. No auditory or reading comprehension; no appropriate verbal or written expression.

1 Severe dysphasia/aphasia. Some auditory and/or reading comprehension at one key word level. May have some verbal or written expression, used occasionally.

2 Severe/moderate dysphasia/aphasia. Auditory and/or reading comprehension consistent with simple commands. Some verbal and/or written expression is used consistently.

3 Moderate dysphasia/aphasia. Auditory and/or reading comprehension is consistent at three word level but is inconsistent with complex commands/structures. May have a specific difficulty in one modality.

4 Mild dysphasia/aphasia. Occasional difficulties present in auditory and/or reading comprehension, and verbal and/or written language.

5 No significant dysphasia/aphasia.

Disability

0 No functional communication. Unable to communicate basic needs. No effective understanding even in context.

1 Minimal communication with maximal assistance and reliant on a "trained listener" such as a familiar person.

2 Occasional effective communication with others, which is helped by context/cues.

3 Consistent communication with others, needs fewer cues and assistance, communication may break down in familiar settings.

4 Occasional difficulties in communicating effectively and requires occasional assistance in some areas or settings.

5 Communicates effectively in all situations.

Handicap

0 No self-confidence/no social integration/not involved in decisions.

1 Low self-confidence/very limited social integration/makes some minor decisions.

2 Some self-confidence/some integration/makes some decisions/in familiar situations.

3 Self-confidence increasing/increasing social integration/makes decisions on aspects of life/in familiar situations.

4 Mostly confident/some difficulties integrating or in fulfilling social role/actively participating in most decisions/may have difficulty in achieving potential in some situations.

5 Confident (appropriate) social role in all situations.

Wellbeing/Distress

0 Severe consistent distress—overt and covert.

1 Severe distress frequently experienced.

2 Moderate consistent distress.

3 Moderate distress frequently experienced.

4 Distress occasionally experienced.

5 No distress (appropriate).

DYSPHASIA/APHASIA

Impairment

0   Severe level of dysphasia/aphasia. Severe dysphasia/aphasia evident in all modalities.
1   Severe/moderate dysphasia/aphasia. Severe dysphasia/aphasia evident in some modalities.
2   Moderate dysphasia/aphasia. Moderate dysphasia/aphasia may have a severe specific difficulty in some areas.
3   Moderate/mild dysphasia/aphasia. Moderate/mild difficulties in some modalities.
4   Mild dysphasia/aphasia. Minimal dysphasia/aphasia present.
5   No dysphasia/aphasia.

Disability

0   No functional communication.
1   Minimal communication with maximal assistance.
2   Some appropriate communication skills helped by cues from a skilled listener.
3   Consistent functional communication with familiar listener.
4   Communicates effectively in most situations, with occasional assistance.
5   Communicates at premorbid level.

Handicap

0   No self-confidence/no social integration/not involved in decisions.
1   Low self-confidence/very limited social integration/makes some minor decisions.
2   Some self-confidence/some integration/makes some decisions/in familiar situations.
3   Self-confidence emerging/integration/makes decisions on aspects of life/in familiar situations.
4   Mostly confident/some difficulties integrating or in fulfilling social role/actively participating most decisions/may have difficulty in achieving potential in some situations.
5   Confident (appropriate) social role in all situations.

Wellbeing/Distress

0   Severe consistent distress—overt and covert.
1   Severe distress frequently experienced.
2   Moderate consistent distress.
3   Moderate distress frequently experienced.
4   Distress occasionally experienced.
5   No distress (appropriate).

APPENDIX C

Pilot Guidance Notes for Outcome Measures Data Form

Pilot Guidance Notes for Outcome Measures Data

1. **Patient's name or identifying code number**
   We do not necessarily require the patient's name. However it would be helpful if you could use a method of identifying clients. This means that in the event that we have difficulty with interpreting the information, and need to get back to you, we can detail the form in the way that you identified the client. This information will not be stored on computer.

2. **Therapy Profession**
   Please detail which therapy profession you belong to. Data will be analyzed by profession.

3. **NHS District/Trust**
   Please identify the Authority/Trust for which you work.

4. **Age**
   Please detail the age of the patient when you recorded their admission score (see point 9 below). Record years, or fraction of years for young children.

5. **Duration of Treatment**
   Detail the duration of treatment in months.

6. **Number of Contacts**
   Detail the amount of attention you have given to a patient. These may be attendances or time spent in influencing care, e.g., discussions with the family etc. A rough guide to your involvement is all that is needed, e.g., 2 attendances +1 chat with relatives +1 chat with nurse in charge = 4.

7. **Locality**
   Please tick the area in which the patient is treated. You can tick more than one of these boxes if the patient's locality changes during the recorded treatment.

8. **Carer**
   Please detail the person "if any" who has assisted with the agreement score (i.e. anybody other than the patient themselves.)

9. **Client Care Group/Etiology/Impairment**
   Please refer to the list of groups appropriate for your therapy profession. Please write down the relevant number code and letter (if applicable), not the names of the aetiologies and impairments.

10. **Ratings**
    A **Admission.** Detail the Outcome Score of the patient when you are first starting treatment. Circle any of the scores that you are aiming to "treat". This row of scores will not have an agreement rating.
    P **Prediction.** Predict an anticipated outcome score and enter a second line of Outcome Scales. This line does not require circling of outcomes worked on or an agreement rating.
    I **Intermediate.** If you alter treatment or have ended an episode of care but without discharging the patient, gauge an Outcome Score and code appropriately. Record an agreement rating of "Complete", "Partial" or "None".
    F **Final.** Rate the ultimate outcome at discharge from the therapy session/service Circling scores on this row is not applicable. Record an agreement rating as above.

Select the score most closely representing your patient's ability. Remember they do not have to be exactly as the descriptor suggests. The descriptors are to help gauge the relative degree of IDHW. Half points (e.g., 2.5) indicate if you think a person is slightly better or worse than a particular score point.

SAMPLE

OUTCOME MEASURES CLIENT DETAIL
SPEECH AND LANGUAGE THERAPY

(1) Patient Name or Identifying Code Number
James Bond 007

(2) Therapy Profession *SPEECH*
(Speech, Physio, Chiropody, Diet, O.T.)

(3) Service Provider *ST. ELSEWHERES*

Patient Details

(4) Age *34* (Years)
(5) Duration of Treatment *6* (Months)
(6) No. of Contacts *21*

(7) Locality
Check appropriate box
☐ Inpatient
☑ Outpatient
☐ Community

(8) Caregiver *SPOUSE*
(Spouse, Mother, etc.)

(9) Client Care Group
Check appropriate box
appropriate box
Please tick one only
☐ Child
☑ Adult *3*

(10) Etiology Code
(See overleaf for codes)
C

(11) Communication Code 1
(See overleaf for codes)
4

Communication Code 2
(as above)
6

(12) Ratings

Code*	(13) Impairment Imp1	Imp2	Disability	Handicap	(14) Wellbeing/Director Patient	Caregiver	Agreement	Date of Rating
A	1	3	2	3	3	2	NA	12/06/95
I	3	3	3.5	4	4	3	2	06/09/95
F	3.5	3	4	4	4	4	3	08/09/95

* A = Admission, I = Intermediate, F = Final.

(15) Comments _____

Note: You may wish to adapt this data collection form to suit your existing patient data system.

APPENDIX D

Pilot Outcome Measures Client Details

Pilot Outcome Measures Client Details

Patient Name or Identifying Code Number

Therapy Profession ....
(Speech, Physio, Chiropody, Diet, O.T)

NHS District/Trust ....

Patient Details

Age ....   Duration of Treatment ....   No. of Contacts ....
(Years)   (Months)

Locality: ☐ In-Patient   Carer ....
Tick appropriate box ☐ Out-Patient   (Spouse, Mother, etc.)
                   ☐ Community

Client Care Group   Etiology Code   Impairment Code
Tick appropriate box ☐ Child   (See overleaf for your codes)   (See overleaf for your codes)
Tick appropriate box ☐ Adult
                                     ....

Ratings
(Remember to circle the outcomes you are working on at each stage)

Code *Type	Impairment	Disability	Handicap	Well-being/ Distress	Agreement	Date of Rating
A					N.A.	/ /
						/ /
						/ /
						/ /
						/ /
						/ /

*A = Admission   P=Prediction   I=Intermediate   F=Final

Comment...
....

Please return to Pam Enderby, Speech Therapy Research Unit
Frenchay Hospital, Bristol, BS16 1LE
Tel. 0272 701212   Fax. 0272 701119

Pilot study   Version 6

Pilot

Speech Therapy
Accepted Etiologies and Impairments

Etiology Groups
1. Mental Illness
2. Cardiovascular
3. Acquired Neurological
   - a. Guillain Barré
   - b. C.V.A.
   - c. Head Injury
   - d. Dementia
   - e. Other
4. Neurosurgery (brain)
5. Orofacial/Neck Surgery
6. Progressive Neurological Disease
   - a. M.S.
   - b. P.D.
   - c. M.N.D.
   - d. Muscular Dystrophy
   - e. Other
7. Voice Pathology
   - a. Structural
   - b. Misuse
   - c. Functional
   - d. Other
8. Burns/Plastics
9. Developmental Delay
10. Cerebral Palsy
11. Hearing Disorders
12. Multifactorial
13. Nothing Abnormal Detected
14. Syndromes
15. Other (please specify)

Communication Codes
1. Disorders of fluency
2. Disorders of voice
3. Laryngectomy
4. Acquired language disorder (Dysphasia)
5. Dyslexia
6. Acquired speech disorder (Dysarthria)
7. Dyspraxia
8. Dysphagia
9. Autism
10. Developmental disorder of language
11. Articulation Impairment
12. Phonological Impairment
13. Deaf Speech/Language
14. Cleft palate speech
15. Learning disability
16. Other (please specify)

APPENDIX E

Validity/Acceptability Check Form

Validity/Acceptability Check Form

You have been identified as a therapist who returned quite a number of outcome forms relating to the pilot project. We appreciate your efforts and would be particularly interested in your views about this method.

I would be grateful if you could answer the following two questions and add any further comments. Please return this form, anonymously, to the address below.

Thanking you for your continued assistance.

----

1. Are the concepts of Impairment, Disability, Handicap and Well Being relevant to Speech and Lanugage Therapy?

    Yes ☐

    No ☐

    If no, please state why

    ....

    ....

    Other comments

    ....

    ....

2. Do you think this approach will be able to reflect the changes you see in your patients?

    ....

    ....

Please state your specialty area   ....

3. Comments: Please add any further comments overleaf.

To: Dr. Pam Enderby : Director
     Speech & Language Therapy Research Unit

APPENDIX F

Speech Therapy Outcomes for Site 1

OVERALL VIEW

TOTAL NUMBER OF PATIENTS = 148

	I	D	H	W
START	2.63	2.48	2.81	3.08
CHANGE	0.83	1.23	1.06	0.99
FINISH	3.46	3.7	3.87	4.07

	% CHANGE IN I	NUMBER OF NO CHANGE	% CHANGE IN D	NUMBER OF NO CHANGE	% CHANGE IN H	NUMBER OF NO CHANGE	% CHANGE IN W	NUMBER OF NO CHANGE
ALL PATIENTS (148)	16.6	45	24.6	27	21.2	46	19.8	63

BY IMPAIRMENT

DISORDER	% CHANGE IN I	NUMBER OF NO CHANGE	% CHANGE IN D	NUMBER OF NO CHANGE	% CHANGE IN H	NUMBER OF NO CHANGE	% CHANGE IN W	NUMBER OF NO CHANGE
DISORDERS OF FLUENCY (8)	1.2	2	7.4	1	20	2	28.6	2
DISORDERS OF VOICE (17)	30.4	4	26.4	3	19.4	5	29.4	4
ACQUIRED LANGUAGE DISORDER (17)	21.6	4	28.2	3	32.2	4	31	6
ACQUIRED SPEECH DISORDER (11)	2.6	8	20	3	5.4	7	8	9
DYSPRAXIA (2)	15	6	35	2	20	1	20	6
DYSPHAGIA (25)	29.2	5	46.6	3	47	8	34.4	12
DEVELOPMENTAL DISORDER OF LANGUAGE (26)	17.8	7	25	6	15.2	15	11.8	19
PHONOLOGICAL IMPAIRMENT (31)	11.6	4	16.4	4	7.4	1	4.4	2
DEAF SPEECH/ LANGUAGE (5)	4	3	4	2	24	2	20	2
LEARNING DISABILITY/ MENTAL RETARDATION (3)	−33.2	0	−23.2	0	−6.6	0	6.6	0

BY IMPAIRMENT

DISORDER	I	D	H	W
DISORDERS OF FLUENCY (8)				
START	3.75	3.56	3	2.75
CHANGE	0.06	0.37	1	1.43
FINISH	3.81	3.93	4	4.18
DISORDERS OF VOICE (17)				
START	2.88	2.94	3.29	2.88
CHANGE	1.52	1.32	0.97	1.47
FINISH	4.41	4.26	4.26	4.35
LARYNGECTOMY (0)				
START				
CHANGE		NO PATIENTS		
FINISH				
ACQUIRED LANGUAGE DISORDER (17) (DYSPHASIA/APHASIA)				
START	2.23	2.35	2.61	2.76
CHANGE	1.08	1.41	1.61	1.55
FINISH	3.32	3.76	4.23	4.32
DYSLEXIA (0)				
START				
CHANGE		NO PATIENTS		
FINISH				
ACQUIRED SPEECH DISORDER (11) (DYSARTHRIA)				
START	2.13	2.72	4	3.5
CHANGE	0.13	1	0.27	0.4
FINISH	2.27	3.72	4.27	3.9
DYSPRAXIA (2)				
START	1	1	1.5	1.5
CHANGE	0.75	1.75	1	1
FINISH	1.75	2.75	2.5	2.5
DYSPHAGIA (25)				
START	2.56	1.88	1.84	2.72
CHANGE	1.46	2.33	2.35	1.72
FINISH	4.02	4.21	4.19	4.44
AUTISM (0)				
START				
CHANGE		NO PATIENTS		
FINISH				
DEVELOPMENTAL DISORDER OF LANGUAGE (26)				
START	2.48	2.01	2.51	3.11
CHANGE	0.89	1.25	0.76	0.59
FINISH	3.38	3.26	3.28	3.71

(continued)

DISORDER	I	D	H	W
ARTICULATION IMPAIRMENT (0)				
START				
CHANGE		NO PATIENTS		
FINISH				
PHONOLOGICAL IMPAIRMENT (31)				
START	3.22	2.9	3.58	4.01
CHANGE	0.58	0.82	0.37	0.22
FINISH	3.8	3.72	3.95	4.24
DEAF SPEECH/LANGUAGE (5)				
START	0.8	1.8	1.2	1.6
CHANGE	0.2	0.2	1.2	1
FINISH	1	2	2.4	2.6
CLEFT PALATE SPEECH (0)				
START				
CHANGE		NO PATIENTS		
FINISH				
LEARNING DISABILITY/				
MENTAL RETARDATION (3)				
START	3.33	3.16	2.33	2.83
CHANGE	− 1.66	− 1.16	− 0.33	0.33
FINISH	1.66	2	2	3.16
OTHERS (0)				
START				
CHANGE		NO PATIENTS		
FINISH				

BY ETIOLOGY

ETIOLOGY	% CHANGE IN I	NUMBER OF NO CHANGE	% CHANGE IN D	NUMBER OF NO CHANGE	% CHANGE IN H	NUMBER OF NO CHANGE	% CHANGE IN W	NUMBER OF NO CHANGE
CARDIOVASCULAR DISEASE (16)	17.4	4	32.4	0	41.2	0	37.4	3
ACQUIRED NEURO-LOGICAL (32)	25.8	9	35.6	8	33	6	24.2	13
NEURO-SURGERY (1)	20	0	20	0	20	0	40	0
PROGRESSIVE NEUROLOGICAL DISEASE (6)	−1.6	5	28.2	1	0	6	0	6
VOICE PATHOLOGY (15)	36	2	29.2	2	22.6	4	36	2
DEVELOPMENTAL DELAY (11)	13.6	2	28	1	18	2	16.2	3
CEREBRAL PALSY (1)	0	1	20	0	0	1	0	1
NOTHING ABNORMAL DETECTED (48)	12	11	17.6	7	12.4	18	10.8	25
SYNDROMES (1)	0	1	20	0	0	1	0	1
OTHERS (5)	10	2	20	2	28	3	32	3

BY ETIOLOGY

ETIOLOGY	I	D	H	W
MENTAL ILLNESS (0)				
START				
CHANGE		NO PATIENTS		
FINISH				
CARDIOVASCULAR DISEASE (16)				
START	3.12	2.56	2.06	2.62
CHANGE	0.87	1.62	2.06	1.87
FINISH	4	4.18	4.12	4.5
ACQUIRED NEUROLOGICAL (32)				
START	2.28	2.18	2.48	2.93
CHANGE	1.29	1.78	1.65	1.21
FINISH	3.57	3.96	4.14	4.15
NEUROSURGERY (1)				
START	3	3	3	2
CHANGE	1	1	1	2
FINISH	4	4	4	4
OROFACIAL/NECK SURGERY (0)				
START				
CHANGE		NO PATIENTS		
FINISH				
PROGRESSIVE NEUROLOGICAL DISEASE (6)				
START	1.08	1.83	4.16	3.41
CHANGE	-0.08	1.41	0	0
FINISH	1	3.25	4.16	3.41
VOICE PATHOLOGY (15)				
START	2.66	2.8	3.2	2.73
CHANGE	1.8	1.46	1.13	1.8
FINISH	4.46	4.26	4.33	4.53
BURNS/PLASTICS (0)				
START				
CHANGE		NO PATIENTS		
FINISH				
DEVELOPMENTAL DELAY (11)				
START	3.09	2.36	2.72	3
CHANGE	0.68	1.4	0.9	0.81
FINISH	3.77	3.77	3.63	3.81
CEREBRAL PALSY (1)				
START	1	2	5	5
CHANGE	0	1	0	0
FINISH	1	3	5	5

(continued)

(continued)

ETIOLOGY	I	D	H	W
HEARING DISORDERS (0)				
START				
CHANGE		NO PATIENTS		
FINISH				
MULTIFACTORIAL (0)				
START				
CHANGE		NO PATIENTS		
FINISH				
NOTHING ABNORMAL DETECTED (48)				
START	3.02	2.67	3.12	3.53
CHANGE	0.6	0.88	0.62	0.54
FINISH	3.62	3.56	3.75	4.07
SYNDROMES (1)				
START	2	1	3	5
CHANGE	0	1	0	0
FINISH	2	2	3	5
OTHERS (5)				
START	2.9	2.7	2.4	2.9
CHANGE	0.5	1	1.4	1.6
FINISH	3.4	3.7	3.8	4.5

APPENDIX G

Speech Therapy Outcomes
for Site 2

OVERALL VIEW

TOTAL NUMBER OF PATIENTS = 335

	I	D	H	W
START	1.84	2.11	1.98	3.02
CHANGE	0.15	0.24	0.23	0.11
FINISH	2	2.36	2.22	3.14

	% CHANGE IN I	NUMBER OF NO CHANGE	% CHANGE IN D	NUMBER OF NO CHANGE	% CHANGE IN H	NUMBER OF NO CHANGE	% CHANGE IN W	NUMBER OF NO CHANGE
ALL PATIENTS (335)	3	252	4.8	210	4.6	210	2.2	266

BY IMPAIRMENT

DISORDER	% CHANGE IN I	NUMBER OF NO CHANGE	% CHANGE IN D	NUMBER OF NO CHANGE	% CHANGE IN H	NUMBER OF NO CHANGE	% CHANGE IN W	NUMBER OF NO CHANGE
DISORDERS OF FLUENCY (3)	3.2	2	3.8	1	0	3	0	3
DISORDERS OF VOICE (2)	5	1	0	2	0	2	10	1
LARYNGECTOMY (0)			NO PATIENTS					
ACQUIRED LANGUAGE DISORDER (2)	5	1	10	0	0	2	0	2
DYSLEXIA (3)	6.6	1	0	3	0	3	20	1
ACQUIRED SPEECH DISORDER (1)	10	0	10	0	0	1	0	1
DYSPRAXIA (2)	0	2	10	0	15	0	5	1
DYSPHAGIA (2)	0	2	5	1	5	1	5	1
AUTISM (9)	5.4	5	7.6	4	5.4	5	1	7
DEVELOPMENTAL DISORDER OF LANGUAGE (22)	5.8	14	7.6	12	6.8	12	0.4	18
ARTICULATION IMPAIRMENT (0)			NO PATIENTS					
PHONOLOGICAL IMPAIRMENT (6)	0.2	5	0	6	0	6	1.6	5
DEAF SPEECH/LANGUAGE (4)	5	3	12.4	1	5	3	10	2
CLEFT PALATE SPEECH (2)	5	1	0	2	0	2	–0	2
LEARNING DISABILITY/MENTAL RETARDATION (275)	2.8	213	4.4	178	4.6	169	2.2	220
OTHERS (1)	0	1	10	0	0	1	0	1

BY IMPAIRMENT

DISORDER	I	D	H	W
DISORDERS OF FLUENCY (3)				
START	2.83	3.33	3.33	3
CHANGE	0.16	0.19	0	0
FINISH	3	3.53	3.33	3
DISORDERS OF VOICE (2)				
START	1.5	2.5	2.25	2
CHANGE	0.25	0	0	0.5
FINISH	1.75	2.5	2.25	2.5
LARYNGECTOMY (0)				
START				
CHANGE		NO PATIENTS		
FINISH				
ACQUIRED LANGUAGE DISORDER (2) (DYSPHASIA/APHASIA)				
START	0.75	0.75	1	4.25
CHANGE	0.25	0.5	0	0
FINISH	1	1.25	1	4.25
DYSLEXIA (3)				
START	1.66	5	3	2.33
CHANGE	0.33	0	0	1
FINISH	2	5	3	3.33
ACQUIRED SPEECH DISORDER (1) (DYSARTHRIA)				
START	3	3	3	3
CHANGE	0.5	0.5	0	0
FINISH	3.5	3.5	3	3
DYSPRAXIA (2)				
START	2	2.5	1.5	3
CHANGE	0	0.5	0.75	0.25
FINISH	2	3	2.25	3.25
DYSPHAGIA (2)				
START	1.25	2	1.5	2
CHANGE	0	0.25	0.25	0.25
FINISH	1.25	2.25	1.75	2.25
AUTISM (9)				
START	0.61	0.83	0.61	1.16
CHANGE	0.27	0.38	0.27	0.05
FINISH	0.88	1.22	0.88	1.22
DEVELOPMENTAL DISORDER OF LANGUAGE (22)				
START	1.56	1.86	1.61	2.38
CHANGE	0.29	0.38	0.34	0.02
FINISH	1.86	2.25	1.95	2.4

(continued)

DISORDER	I	D	H	W
ARTICULATION IMPAIRMENT (0)				
START				
CHANGE		NO PATIENTS		
FINISH				
PHONOLOGICAL IMPAIRMENT (6)				
START	2.33	2.66	2.75	3
CHANGE	0.01	0	0	0.08
FINISH	2.35	2.66	2.75	3.08
DEAF SPEECH/LANGUAGE (4)				
START	2	2	2.25	2.5
CHANGE	0.25	0.62	0.25	0.5
FINISH	2.25	2.62	2.5	3
CLEFT PALATE SPEECH (2)				
START	2.5	3	3	3
CHANGE	0.25	0	0	− 0.25
FINISH	2.75	3	3	2.75
LEARNING DISABILITY/ MENTAL RETARDATION (275)				
START	1.88	2.11	2.01	3.16
CHANGE	0.14	0.22	0.23	0.11
FINISH	2.03	2.34	2.24	3.27
OTHERS (1)				
START	2.5	3	3	3
CHANGE	0	0.5	0	0
FINISH	2.5	3.5	3	3

BY ETIOLOGY

ETIOLOGY	% CHANGE IN I	NUMBER OF NO CHANGE	% CHANGE IN D	NUMBER OF NO CHANGE	% CHANGE IN H	NUMBER OF NO CHANGE	% CHANGE IN W	NUMBER OF NO CHANGE
MENTAL ILLNESS (0)	NO PATIENTS							
CARDIOVASCULAR DISEASE (1)	0	1	20	0	0	1	0	1
ACQUIRED NEURO-LOGICAL (6)	3.2	4	5	3	3.2	5	0	6
NEURO-SURGERY (0)	NO PATIENTS							
OROFACIAL/NECK SURGERY (1)	0	1	10	0	10	0	40	0
PROGRESSIVE NEUROLOGICAL DISEASE (1)	0	1	20	0	0	1	0	1
VOICE PATHOLOGY (2)	5	1	5	1	5	1	5	1
BURNS/PLASTICS (0)	NO PATIENTS							
DEVELOPMENTAL DELAY (64)	3.4	47	6	41	6	38	2.6	56
CEREBRAL PALSY (23)	1.2	19	2	17	2.6	15	-1.6	20
HEARING DISORDERS (0)	NO PATIENTS							
MULTI-FACTORIAL (112)	3.4	86	4.6	73	6	63	3.8	84
NOTHING ABNORMAL DETECTED (1)	0	1	30	0	20	0	-20	1
SYNDROMES (93)	3.6	68	5	55	3.2	64	2.4	71
OTHERS (19)	-0.4	14	3	11	2	12	-6.8	16

BY ETIOLOGY

ETIOLOGY	I	D	H	W
MENTAL ILLNESS (0)				
START				
CHANGE		NO PATIENTS		
FINISH				
CARDIOVASCULAR DISEASE (1)				
START	0	0	0	0
CHANGE	0	1	0	0
FINISH	0	1	0	0
ACQUIRED NEUROLOGICAL (6)				
START	1.41	1.41	1.33	3.66
CHANGE	0.16	0.25	0.16	0
FINISH	1.58	1.66	1.5	3.66
NEUROSURGERY (0)				
START				
CHANGE		NO PATIENTS		
FINISH				
OROFACIAL/NECK SURGERY (1)				
START	3	4	4	1
CHANGE	0	0.5	0.5	2
FINISH	3	4.5	4.5	3
PROGRESSIVE NEUROLOGICAL DISEASE (1)				
START	2	2	3	4
CHANGE	0	1	0	0
FINISH	2	3	3	4
VOICE PATHOLOGY (2)				
START	2.5	3.5	2.5	3.5
CHANGE	0.25	0.25	0.25	0.25
FINISH	2.75	3.75	2.75	3.75
BURNS/PLASTICS (0)				
START				
CHANGE		NO PATIENTS		
FINISH				
DEVELOPMENTAL DELAY (64)				
START	2	2.25	2.05	3.1
CHANGE	0.17	0.3	0.3	0.13
FINISH	2.17	2.56	2.35	3.24
CEREBRAL PALSY (23)				
START	1.78	1.93	1.69	3.41
CHANGE	0.06	0.1	0.13	− 0.08
FINISH	1.84	2.04	1.82	3.32

(continued)

(continued)

ETIOLOGY	I	D	H	W
HEARING DISORDERS (0)				
START				
CHANGE		NO PATIENTS		
FINISH				
MULTIFACTORIAL (112)				
START	1.63	1.89	1.76	2.77
CHANGE	0.17	0.23	0.3	0.19
FINISH	1.8	2.12	2.07	2.96
NOTHING ABNORMAL DETECTED (1)				
START	2.5	2	1	3
CHANGE	0	1.5	1	− 1
FINISH	2.5	3.5	2	2
SYNDROMES (93)				
START	1.98	2.27	2.23	3.23
CHANGE	0.18	0.25	0.16	0.12
FINISH	2.17	2.52	2.39	3.36
OTHERS (19)				
START	2.02	2.05	2.05	3.26
CHANGE	− 0.02	0.15	0.1	− 0.34
FINISH	2	2.21	2.15	2.92

APPENDIX H

Speech Therapy Outcomes
for Site 3

OVERALL VIEW
TOTAL NUMBER OF PATIENTS = 232

	I	D	H	W
START	2.07	2.29	2.21	2.71
CHANGE	0.58	0.69	0.79	0.62
FINISH	2.65	2.99	3.01	3.33

	% CHANGE IN I	NUMBER OF NO CHANGE	% CHANGE IN D	NUMBER OF NO CHANGE	% CHANGE IN H	NUMBER OF NO CHANGE	% CHANGE IN W	NUMBER OF NO CHANGE
ALL PATIENTS (232)	11.6	116	13.8	97	15.8	86	12.4	101

BY IMPAIRMENT

DISORDER	% CHANGE IN I	NUMBER OF NO CHANGE	% CHANGE IN D	NUMBER OF NO CHANGE	% CHANGE IN H	NUMBER OF NO CHANGE	% CHANGE IN W	NUMBER OF NO CHANGE
DISORDERS OF FLUENCY (7)	22.8	3	28.4	2	30	1	34.2	2
DISORDERS OF VOICE (26)	26	8	25.2	7	31.4	5	30.6	3
ACQUIRED LANGUAGE DISORDER (34)	11.6	16	21.4	6	19	10	7.2	17
DYSLEXIA (1)	0	1	0	1	30	0	30	0
ACQUIRED SPEECH DISORDER (2)	10	0	5	1	30	0	30	0
DYSPRAXIA (5)	14	1	12	1	8	2	10	2
DYSPHAGIA (1)	0	1	0	1	0	1	0	1
AUTISM (1)	10	0	10	0	0	1	20	0
DEVELOPMENTAL DISORDER OF LANGUAGE (51)	11.8	24	14.6	20	14.4	20	11	25
PHONOLOGICAL IMPAIRMENT (42)	17.6	9	12.6	20	15.4	20	9	24
DEAF SPEECH/ LANGUAGE (1)	10	0	0	1	10	0	20	0
CLEFT PALATE SPEECH (2)	10	1	10	1	10	1	10	1
LEARNING DISABILITY/ MENTAL RETARDATION (53)	−0.8	49	4	33	8	22	6.8	22
OTHERS (6)	10	3	6.6	3	6.6	3	13.2	4

BY IMPAIRMENT

DISORDER	I	D	H	W
DISORDERS OF FLUENCY (7)				
START	2.14	1.92	1.92	1.85
CHANGE	1.14	1.42	1.5	1.71
FINISH	3.28	3.35	3.42	3.57
DISORDERS OF VOICE (26)				
START	2.42	2.44	2.48	2.23
CHANGE	1.3	1.26	1.57	1.53
FINISH	3.73	3.71	4.05	3.76
LARYNGECTOMY (0)				
START				
CHANGE		NO PATIENTS		
FINISH				
ACQUIRED LANGUAGE DISORDER (34) (DYSPHASIA/APHASIA)				
START	1.47	1.61	1.66	3.04
CHANGE	0.58	1.07	0.95	0.36
FINISH	2.05	2.69	2.61	3.41
DYSLEXIA (1)				
START	3	3	3	3
CHANGE	0	0	1.5	1.5
FINISH	3	3	4.5	4.5
ACQUIRED SPEECH DISORDER (2) (DYSARTHRIA)				
START	3	3.5	2.5	2
CHANGE	0.5	0.25	1.5	1.5
FINISH	3.5	3.75	4	3.5
DYSPRAXIA (5)				
START	1.3	1.5	2	2.4
CHANGE	0.7	0.6	0.4	0.5
FINISH	2	2.09	2.4	2.9
DYSPHAGIA (1)				
START	2	3	3	2
CHANGE	− 1	0	− 1	0
FINISH	1	3	2	2
AUTISM (1)				
START	2	2	2	1
CHANGE	0.5	0.5	0	1
FINISH	2.5	2.5	2	2
DEVELOPMENTAL DISORDER OF LANGUAGE (51)				
START	2.2	2.14	2.24	2.7
CHANGE	0.59	0.73	0.72	0.55
FINISH	2.8	2.88	2.97	3.26

(continued)

DISORDER	I	D	H	W
ARTICULATION IMPAIRMENT (0)				
START				
CHANGE		NO PATIENTS		
FINISH				
PHONOLOGICAL IMPAIRMENT (42)				
START	2.58	3	2.86	3.57
CHANGE	0.88	0.63	0.77	0.45
FINISH	3.46	3.63	3.64	4.02
DEAF SPEECH/LANGUAGE (1)				
START	3	3	2	2
CHANGE	0.5	0	0.5	1
FINISH	3.5	3	2.5	3
CLEFT PALATE SPEECH (2)				
START	2.5	3	3.5	3.5
CHANGE	0.5	0.5	0.5	0.5
FINISH	3	3.5	4	4
LEARNING DISABILITY/				
MENTAL RETARDATION (53)				
START	1.76	2.23	1.87	2.16
CHANGE	− 0.04	0.2	0.4	0.34
FINISH	1.71	2.44	2.28	2.51
OTHERS (6)				
START	1.83	2.66	2.33	3.5
CHANGE	0.5	0.33	0.33	0.66
FINISH	2.33	3	2.66	4.16

BY ETIOLOGY

ETIOLOGY	% CHANGE IN I	NUMBER OF NO CHANGE	% CHANGE IN D	NUMBER OF NO CHANGE	% CHANGE IN H	NUMBER OF NO CHANGE	% CHANGE IN W	NUMBER OF NO CHANGE
ACQUIRED NEUROLOGICAL (38)	11	18	19.6	8	19.4	11	9.6	17
OROFACIAL/NECK SURGERY (3)	20	1	13.2	1	20	1	20	1
PROGRESSIVE NEUROLOGICAL DISEASE (1)	−20	1	0	1	−20	1	0	1
VOICE PATHOLOGY (245)	26.6	7	26.2	7	34	3	32	2
DEVELOPMENTAL DELAY (83)	16.2	25	15.8	33	15.6	36	12	41
CEREBRAL PALSY (1)	0	1	10	0	10	0	0	1
MULTI-FACTORIAL (5)	0	5	0	5	−4	4	8	3
NOTHING ABNORMAL DETECTED (26)	9.2	13	9.2	12	10.2	12	10	14
SYNDROMES (7)	2.8	6	1	6	8.2	2	1.4	6
OTHERS (42)	0	37	5.8	22	9.6	15	8.4	14

BY ETIOLOGY

ETIOLOGY	I	D	H	W
MENTAL ILLNESS (0)				
START				
CHANGE		NO PATIENTS		
FINISH				
CARDIOVASCULAR DISEASE (0)				
START				
CHANGE		NO PATIENTS		
FINISH				
ACQUIRED NEUROLOGICAL (38)				
START	1.65	1.81	1.8	2.96
CHANGE	0.55	0.98	0.97	0.48
FINISH	2.21	2.8	2.77	3.44
NEUROSURGERY (0)				
START				
CHANGE		NO PATIENTS		
FINISH				
OROFACIAL/NECK SURGERY (3)				
START	2.33	2.66	3	3
CHANGE	1	.33	1	1
FINISH	3.33	.66	4	4
PROGRESSIVE NEUROLOGICAL DISEASE (1)				
START	2	3	3	2
CHANGE	−1	0	−1	0
FINISH	1	3	2	2
VOICE PATHOLOGY (24)				
START	2.37	2.31	2.35	2.16
CHANGE	1.33	1.31	1.7	1.6
FINISH	3.7	3.62	4.06	3.77
BURNS/PLASTICS (0)				
START				
CHANGE		NO PATIENTS		
FINISH				
DEVELOPMENTAL DELAY (83)				
START	2.25	2.36	2.39	2.97
CHANGE	0.81	0.79	0.78	0.6
FINISH	3.06	3.16	3.18	3.58
CEREBRAL PALSY (1)				
START	2	2	2	3.5
CHANGE	0	0.5	0.5	0
FINISH	2	2.5	2.5	3.5

(continued)

(continued)

ETIOLOGY	I	D	H	W
HEARING DISORDERS (0)				
START				
CHANGE		NO PATIENTS		
FINISH				
MULTIFACTORIAL (5)				
START	1.4	1.9	1.6	2.3
CHANGE	0	− 0.2	0	0.4
FINISH	1.4	1.7	1.6	2.7
NOTHING ABNORMAL DETECTED (26)				
START	2.42	2.73	2.76	3.03
CHANGE	0.46	0.46	0.51	0.5
FINISH	2.88	3.19	3.28	3.53
SYNDROMES (7)				
START	2.42	2.57	2.5	3.71
CHANGE	0.14	0.05	0.41	0.07
FINISH	2.57	2.62	2.91	3.78
OTHERS (42)				
START	1.66	2.26	1.75	1.88
CHANGE	0	0.29	0.48	0.42
FINISH	1.66	2.55	2.23	2.3

APPENDIX I

Speech Therapy Outcomes for Site 4

OVERALL VIEW
TOTAL NUMBER OF PATIENTS = 70

	I	D	H	W
START	1.8	2.15	2.16	2.57
CHANGE	1.15	1.16	1.17	1.19
FINISH	2.96	3.32	3.33	3.76

	% CHANGE IN I	NUMBER OF NO CHANGE	% CHANGE IN D	NUMBER OF NO CHANGE	% CHANGE IN H	NUMBER OF NO CHANGE	% CHANGE IN W	NUMBER OF NO CHANGE
ALL PATIENTS (70)	23	32	23.2	23	23.4	29	23.8	26

BY IMPAIRMENT

DISORDER	% CHANGE IN I	NUMBER OF NO CHANGE	% CHANGE IN D	NUMBER OF NO CHANGE	% CHANGE IN H	NUMBER OF NO CHANGE	% CHANGE IN W	NUMBER OF NO CHANGE
DISORDERS OF FLUENCY (5)	16	2	40	0	40	0	40	0
DISORDERS OF VOICE (11)	49	0	32.6	1	42.6	0	45.4	0
ACQUIRED LANGUAGE DISORDER (9)	32.2	0	25.4	2	31	2	35.4	1
DYSPHAGIA (6)	73.2	0	70	0	66.6	1	56.6	0
DEVELOPMENTAL DISORDER OF LANGUAGE (1)	0	1	0	1	0	1	0	1
PHONOLOGICAL IMPAIRMENT (13)	16	7	10	9	6	12	7.6	10
LEARNING DISABILITY (21)	1.8	19	12.8	7	9	11	8.4	12
OTHERS (3)	0	3	0	3	0	3	3.2	2

BY IMPAIRMENT

DISORDER	I	D	H	W
DISORDERS OF FLUENCY (5)				
START	2.8	2.4	2.6	2.4
CHANGE	0.8	2	2	2
FINISH	3.6	4.4	4.6	4.4
DISORDERS OF VOICE (11)				
START	1.45	2	1.59	1.54
CHANGE	2.45	1.63	2.13	2.27
FINISH	3.9	3.63	3.72	3.81
LARYNGECTOMY (0)				
START				
CHANGE		NO PATIENTS		
FINISH				
ACQUIRED LANGUAGE DISORDER (9) **(DYSPHASIA/APHASIA)**				
START	1.44	1.5	1.27	2.33
CHANGE	1.61	1.27	1.55	1.77
FINISH	3.05	2.77	2.83	4.11
DYSLEXIA (0)				
START				
CHANGE		NO PATIENTS		
FINISH				
ACQUIRED SPEECH DISORDER (0) **(DYSARTHRIA)**				
START				
CHANGE		NO PATIENTS		
FINISH				
DYSPRAXIA (0)				
START				
CHANGE		NO PATIENTS		
FINISH				
DYSPHAGIA (6)				
START	0.33	0.33	0.66	0.5
CHANGE	3.66	3.5	3.33	2.83
FINISH	4	3.83	4	3.33
AUTISM (0)				
START				
CHANGE		NO PATIENTS		
FINISH				
DEVELOPMENTAL DISORDER OF LANGUAGE (1)				
START	4.5	3.5	1.5	5
CHANGE	0	0	0	0
FINISH	4.5	3.5	1.5	5

(continued)

DISORDER	I	D	H	W
ARTICULATION IMPAIRMENT (0)				
START				
CHANGE		NO PATIENTS		
FINISH				
PHONOLOGICAL IMPAIRMENT (13)				
START	2.5	3.38	4.19	4.15
CHANGE	0.8	0.5	0.3	0.38
FINISH	3.3	3.88	4.5	4.53
DEAF SPEECH/LANGUAGE (0)				
START				
CHANGE		NO PATIENTS		
FINISH				
CLEFT PALATE SPEECH (0)				
START				
CHANGE		NO PATIENTS		
FINISH				
LEARNING DISABILITY/ MENTAL RETARDATION (21)				
START	1.33	1.9	1.76	2.69
CHANGE	0.09	0.64	0.45	0.42
FINISH	1.42	2.54	2.21	3.11
OTHERS (3)				
START	4.83	3.66	2.83	2.5
CHANGE	0	0	0	0.16
FINISH	4.83	3.66	2.83	2.66

BY ETIOLOGY

ETIOLOGY	% CHANGE IN I	NUMBER OF NO CHANGE	% CHANGE IN D	NUMBER OF NO CHANGE	% CHANGE IN H	NUMBER OF NO CHANGE	% CHANGE IN W	NUMBER OF NO CHANGE
ACQUIRED NEURO-LOGICAL (15)	48.6	0	43.2	2	45.2	3	44	1
VOICE PATHOLOGY (11)	49	0	32.6	1	42.6	0	45.4	0
DEVELOPMENTAL DELAY (3)	46.6	0	20	1	0	3	0	3
CEREBRAL PALSY (6)	0	6	0	6	1.6	5	6.6	3
MULTI-FACTORIAL (14)	8.4	9	25.6	1	22	4	20	5
NOTHING ABNORMAL DETECTED (10)	9	6	9	7	10	8	12	6
SYNDROMES (6)	0	6	18.2	0	11.6	2	10	4
OTHERS (4)	0	4	0	4	0	4	2.4	3

BY ETIOLOGY

ETIOLOGY	I	D	H	W
MENTAL ILLNESS (0)				
START				
CHANGE		NO PATIENTS		
FINISH				
CARDIOVASCULAR DISEASE (0)				
START				
CHANGE		NO PATIENTS		
FINISH				
ACQUIRED NEUROLOGICAL (15)				
START	1	1.03	1.03	1.6
CHANGE	2.43	2.16	2.26	2.2
FINISH	3.43	3.2	3.3	3.8
NEUROSURGERY (0)				
START				
CHANGE		NO PATIENTS		
FINISH				
OROFACIAL/NECK SURGERY (0)				
START				
CHANGE		NO PATIENTS		
FINISH				
PROGRESSIVE NEUROLOGICAL DISEASE (0)				
START				
CHANGE		NO PATIENTS		
FINISH				
VOICE PATHOLOGY (11)				
START	1.45	2	1.59	1.54
CHANGE	2.45	1.63	2.13	2.27
FINISH	3.9	3.63	3.72	3.81
BURNS/PLASTICS (0)				
START				
CHANGE		NO PATIENTS		
FINISH				
DEVELOPMENTAL DELAY (3)				
START	1	1.03	1.03	1.6
CHANGE	2.43	2.16	2.26	2.2
FINISH	3.43	3.2	3.3	3.8
CEREBRAL PALSY (6)				
START	1.45	2	1.59	1.54
CHANGE	2.45	1.63	2.13	2.27
FINISH	3.9	3.63	3.72	3.81

(continued)

(continued)

ETIOLOGY	I	D	H	W
HEARING DISORDERS (0)				
START				
CHANGE		NO PATIENTS		
FINISH				
MULTIFACTORIAL (14)				
START	2.66	4	5	5
CHANGE	2.33	1	0	0
FINISH	5	5	5	5
NOTHING ABNORMAL DETECTED (10)				
START	1.16	2.33	2.25	2.91
CHANGE	0	0	0.08	0.33
FINISH	1.16	2.33	2.33	3.25
SYNDROMES (6)				
START	1.83	2	2.25	2.83
CHANGE	0	0.91	0.58	0.5
FINISH	1.83	2.91	2.83	3.33
OTHERS (4)				
START	4.75	3.62	2.5	3.12
CHANGE	0	0	0	0.12
FINISH	4.75	3.62	2.5	3.25

APPENDIX J

Speech Therapy Outcomes
for Site 5

BY IMPAIRMENT

DISORDER	% CHANGE IN I	NUMBER OF NO CHANGE	% CHANGE IN D	NUMBER OF NO CHANGE	% CHANGE IN H	NUMBER OF NO CHANGE	% CHANGE IN W	NUMBER OF NO CHANGE
ACQUIRED LANGUAGE DISORDER (DYSPHASIA/ APHASIA) (8)	22.4	2	25	1	30	3	22.4	1

BY IMPAIRMENT

DISORDER	I	D	H	W
ACQUIRED LANGUAGE DISORDER (DYSPHASIA/APHASIA)				
START	2	1.87	1.87	3
CHANGE	1.12	1.25	1.5	1.12
FINISH	3.12	3.12	3.37	4.12

BY ETIOLOGY

ETIOLOGY	% CHANGE IN I	NUMBER OF NO CHANGE	% CHANGE IN D	NUMBER OF NO CHANGE	% CHANGE IN H	NUMBER OF NO CHANGE	% CHANGE IN W	NUMBER OF NO CHANGE
ACQUIRED NEUROLOGICAL (7)	22.8	2	25.6	1	28.4	3	22.8	1
PROGRESSIVE NEUROLOGICAL DISEASE (1)	20	0	20	0	40	0	20	0

BY ETIOLOGY

ETIOLOGY	I	D	H	W
ACQUIRED NEUROLOGICAL (7)				
START	1.71	1.57	1.71	2.85
CHANGE	1.14	1.28	1.42	1.14
FINISH	2.85	2.85	3.14	4
PROGRESSIVE NEUROLOGICAL DISEASE (1)				
START	4	4	3	4
CHANGE	1	1	2	1
FINISH	5	5	5	5

APPENDIX K

Speech Therapy Outcomes
for Site 6

OVERALL VIEW
TOTAL NUMBER OF PATIENTS = 65

	I	D	H	W
START	2.32	2.39	1.59	2.22
CHANGE	0.72	0.66	0.67	0.47
FINISH	3.05	3.05	2.27	2.7

	% CHANGE IN I	NUMBER OF NO CHANGE	% CHANGE IN D	NUMBER OF NO CHANGE	% CHANGE IN H	NUMBER OF NO CHANGE	% CHANGE IN W	NUMBER OF NO CHANGE
ALL PATIENTS (65)	18.6	19	18.2	24	15.6	27	16.6	27

BY IMPAIRMENT

DISORDER	% CHANGE IN I	NUMBER OF NO CHANGE	% CHANGE IN D	NUMBER OF NO CHANGE	% CHANGE IN H	NUMBER OF NO CHANGE	% CHANGE IN W	NUMBER OF NO CHANGE
OVERALL (65)	18.6	19	18.2	24	15.6	27	16.6	27
DISORDERS OF VOICE (6)	48.6	0	42.4	0	36.2	1	38.6	1
DYSPHASIA/ APHASIA (20)	12.2	5	10.4	8	21	4	12.6	8
DYSARTHRIA (1)	0	1	20	0	20	0	60	0
DYSPHAGIA (24)	17.2	7	16.4	11	6	16	6	15
AUTISM (1)	0	1	0	1	0	1	0	1
DEVELOPMENTAL DISORDER OF LANGUAGE (6)	15	2	13.2	2	16.6	1	20	0
LEARNING DISABILITY (3)	6	2	20	1	10	3	32	1

BY IMPAIRMENT

DISORDER	I	D	H	W
OVERALL (65)				
START	2.04	2.19	1.9	2
CHANGE	0.93	0.91	0.78	0.83
FINISH	2.97	3.1	2.68	2.83
DISORDERS OF VOICE (8)				
START	1.87	2.06	2.62	1.75
CHANGE	2.43	2.12	1.81	1.93
FINISH	4.31	4.18	4.43	3.68
DYSPHASIA/APHASIA (20)				
START	2.27	2.25	1.27	1.91
CHANGE	0.61	0.52	1.05	0.63
FINISH	2.88	2.77	2.33	2.55
DYSARTHRIA (1)				
START	2	2	1	0
CHANGE	0	1	1	3
FINISH	2	3	2	3
DYSPHAGIA (24)				
START	2.43	2.69	2.17	2.65
CHANGE	0.86	0.82	0.3	0.3
FINISH	3.3	3.52	2.47	2.95
AUTISM (1)				
START	1	1	1	1
CHANGE	0	0	0	0
FINISH	1	1	1	1
DEVELOPMENTAL DISORDER OF LANGUAGE (6)				
START	1.41	1.83	2.16	2
CHANGE	0.75	0.66	0.83	1
FINISH	2.16	2.5	3	3
LEARNING DISABILITY (5)				
START	1.1	1.1	2.09	0.7
CHANGE	0.3	1	0.5	1.6
FINISH	1.4	2.09	2.6	2.3

BY ETIOLOGY

ETIOLOGY	% CHANGE IN I	NUMBER OF NO CHANGE	% CHANGE IN D	NUMBER OF NO CHANGE	% CHANGE IN H	NUMBER OF NO CHANGE	% CHANGE IN W	NUMBER OF NO CHANGE
OVERALL (65)	18.6	19	18.2	24	15.6	27	16.6	27
ACQUIRED NEURO-LOGICAL (37)	14.4	11	13.2	17	13.4	17	9.4	20
NEURO-SURGERY (1)	20	0	40	0	20	0	0	1
OROFACIAL/NECK SURGERY (1)	60	0	60	0	20	0	40	0
PROGRESSIVE NEUROLOGICAL DISEASE (2)	20	1	20	0	10	1	30	1
VOICE PATHOLOGY (8)	48.6	0	42.4	0	36.2	1	38.6	1
CEREBRAL PALSY (2)	0	1	5	1	20	0	10	1
NOTHING ABNORMAL DETECTED (7)	14.2	3	18.4	3	17	2	22.8	1
SYNDROMES (3)	0	2	10	1	3.2	2	20	1
OTHERS (4)	12.4	1	12.4	2	0	4	20	1

BY ETIOLOGY

ETIOLOGY	I	D	H	W
OVERALL (65)				
START	2.32	2.39	1.59	2.22
CHANGE	0.72	0.66	0.67	0.47
FINISH	3.05	3.05	2.27	2.27
ACQUIRED NEUROLOGICAL (37)				
START	2.32	2.39	1.59	2.22
CHANGE	0.72	0.66	0.67	0.47
FINISH	3.05	3.05	2.27	2.7
NEUROSURGERY (1)				
START	2	2	2	3
CHANGE	1	2	1	0
FINISH	3	4	3	3
OROFACIAL/NECK SURGERY (1)				
START	0	0	1	0
CHANGE	3	3	1	2
FINISH	3	3	2	2
PROGRESSIVE NEUROLOGICAL DISEASE (2)				
START	2.5	3	1.5	1.5
CHANGE	1	1	0.5	1.5
FINISH	3.5	4	2	3
VOICE PATHOLOGY (8)				
START	1.87	2.06	2.62	1.75
CHANGE	2.43	2.12	1.81	1.93
FINISH	4.31	4.18	4.43	3.68
CEREBRAL PALSY (2)				
START	1.5	1	2	2.5
CHANGE	0.25	0.25	1	0.5
FINISH	1.75	1.25	3	3
NOTHING ABNORMAL DETECTED (7)				
START	1.21	1.71	2	1.71
CHANGE	0.71	0.92	0.85	1.41
FINISH	1.92	2.64	2.85	2.85
SYNDROMES (3)				
START	1.5	1.33	2.16	0.83
CHANGE	0	0.5	0.16	1
FINISH	1.5	1.83	2.32	1.83
OTHERS (4)				
START	2.25	2.87	3.25	2
CHANGE	0.62	0.62	0	1
FINISH	2.87	3.5	3.25	3

APPENDIX L

Speech Therapy Outcomes for Site 7

OVERALL VIEW
TOTAL NUMBER OF PATIENTS = 290

	I	D	H	W
START	2.11	2.52	2.41	2.78
CHANGE	0.44	0.53	0.55	0.53
FINISH	2.55	3.06	2.96	3.31

	% CHANGE IN I	NUMBER OF NO CHANGE	% CHANGE IN D	NUMBER OF NO CHANGE	% CHANGE IN H	NUMBER OF NO CHANGE	% CHANGE IN W	NUMBER OF NO CHANGE
ALL PATIENTS (290)	8.8	175	10.6	140	11	149	10.6	165

BY IMPAIRMENT

DISORDER	% CHANGE IN I	NUMBER OF NO CHANGE	% CHANGE IN D	NUMBER OF NO CHANGE	% CHANGE IN H	NUMBER OF NO CHANGE	% CHANGE IN W	NUMBER OF NO CHANGE
DISORDERS OF FLUENCY (9)	18.8	5	14.4	4	21	3	31	1
DISORDERS OF VOICE (17)	19.4	2	18.2	3	20	7	23.4	3
LARYNGECTOMY (0)			NO PATIENTS					
ACQUIRED LANGUAGE DISORDER (11)	7.2	5	12.6	3	14.4	6	-2.6	7
DYSLEXIA (0)			NO PATIENTS					
ACQUIRED SPEECH DISORDER (4)	2.4	3	5	3	22.4	1	15	2
DYSPRAXIA/APRAXIA (4)	5	3	12.4	2	0	4	7.4	2
DYSPHAGIA (8)	-2.4	7	0	5	2.4	6	11.2	3
AUTISM (11)	0.8	10	10	5	5.4	7	9	5
DEVELOPMENTAL DISORDER OF LANGUAGE (70)	17	25	17.4	23	15.4	27	16.4	31
ARTICULATION IMPAIRMENT (0)			NO PATIENTS					
PHONOLOGICAL IMPAIRMENT (56)	10.8	23	8.2	30	10	30	7.2	39
DEAF SPEECH/LANGUAGE (3)	3.2	2	3.2	2	16.6	0	13.2	1
CLEFT PALATE SPEECH (1)	40	0	40	0	40	0	60	0
LEARNING DISABILITY/MENTAL RETARDATION (83)	0	81	5	54	6.2	50	4.2	62
OTHERS (4)	5	3	12.4	1	2.4	3	7.4	2

BY IMPAIRMENT

DISORDER	I	D	H	W
DISORDERS OF FLUENCY (9)				
START	2.38	2.83	2.44	1.88
CHANGE	0.94	0.72	1.05	1.55
FINISH	3.33	3.55	3.5	3.44
DISORDERS OF VOICE (17)				
START	2.61	3.02	3.29	2.82
CHANGE	0.97	0.91	1	1.17
FINISH	3.58	3.94	4.29	4
LARYNGECTOMY (0)				
START				
CHANGE		NO PATIENTS		
FINISH				
ACQUIRED LANGUAGE DISORDER (DYSPHASIA/APHASIA) (11)				
START	1.72	2	1.72	2.9
CHANGE	0.36	0.63	0.72	−0.13
FINISH	2.09	2.63	2.44	2.77
DYSLEXIA (0)				
START				
CHANGE		NO PATIENTS		
FINISH				
ACQUIRED SPEECH DISORDER (DYSARTHRIA) (4)				
START	1.75	3.25	2	2.75
CHANGE	0.12	0.25	1.12	0.75
FINISH	1.87	3.5	3.12	3.5
DYSPRAXIA/APRAXIA (4)				
START	1.75	3	3.12	3.5
CHANGE	0.25	0.62	0	0.37
FINISH	2	3.62	3.12	3.87
DYSPHAGIA (8)				
START	2.25	2.43	1.37	2.75
CHANGE	−0.12	0	0.12	0.56
FINISH	2.12	2.43	1.5	3.31
AUTISM (11)				
START	1.31	1.81	1.5	1.72
CHANGE	0.04	0.5	0.27	0.45
FINISH	1.36	2.31	1.77	2.18
DEVELOPMENTAL DISORDER OF LANGUAGE (70)				
START	1.85	2.15	2.21	2.71
CHANGE	0.85	0.87	0.77	0.82
FINISH	2.71	3.02	2.99	3.54

(continued)

DISORDER	I	D	H	W
ARTICULATION IMPAIRMENT (0)				
START				
CHANGE		NO PATIENTS		
FINISH				
PHONOLOGICAL IMPAIRMENT (56)				
START	2.72	3.02	3.03	3.49
CHANGE	0.54	0.41	0.5	0.36
FINISH	3.26	3.43	3.54	3.85
DEAF SPEECH/LANGUAGE (3)				
START	1.33	1.66	1.66	2
CHANGE	0.16	0.16	0.83	0.66
FINISH	1.5	1.83	2.5	2.66
CLEFT PALATE SPEECH (1)				
START	0	1	1	0
CHANGE	2	2	2	3
FINISH	2	3	3	3
LEARNING DISABILITY/ MENTAL RETARDATION (83)				
START	1.98	2.5	2.28	2.56
CHANGE	0	0.25	0.31	0.21
FINISH	1.98	2.75	2.59	2.78
OTHERS (4)				
START	2.5	3	2.75	3.75
CHANGE	0.25	0.62	0.12	0.37
FINISH	2.75	3.62	2.87	4.12

BY ETIOLOGY

ETIOLOGY	% CHANGE IN I	NUMBER OF NO CHANGE	% CHANGE IN D	NUMBER OF NO CHANGE	% CHANGE IN H	NUMBER OF NO CHANGE	% CHANGE IN W	NUMBER OF NO CHANGE
MENTAL ILLNESS (0)	NO PATIENTS							
CARDIOVASCULAR DISEASE (4)	10	2	20	1	15	1	15	2
ACQUIRED NEURO-LOGICAL (12)	10.8	5	15	4	15.8	6	7.4	5
NEUROSURGERY (0)			NO PATIENTS					
OROFACIAL/NECK SURGERY (1)	0	1	0	1	20	0	20	0
PROGRESSIVE NEUROLOGICAL (3)	-13.2	2	-13.2	2	0	3	-20	2
VOICE PATHOLOGY (16)	18.6	2	18	3	21.2	6	25	2
BURNS/PLASTICS (1)	0	1	10	0	0	1	0	1
DEVELOPMENTAL DELAY (113)	7.6	64	8.6	60	9.4	62	5.6	77
CEREBRAL PALSY (8)	0	8	5	6	10	4	10	6
HEARING DISORDERS (0)			NO PATIENTS					
MULTI-FACTORIAL (42)	-7.4	3	-12.4	3	-5	4	0	3
NOTHING ABNORMAL DETECTED (53)	21.4	19	18.6	17	18.2	16	24	20
SYNDROMES (21)	2.8	19	7.6	13	7	14	6.6	16
OTHERS (48)	2.4	42	8.8	25	6	30	7.4	28

BY ETIOLOGY

ETIOLOGY	I	D	H	W
MENTAL ILLNESS (0)				
START				
CHANGE		NO PATIENTS		
FINISH				
CARDIOVASCULAR DISEASE (4)				
START	1.5	1.75	1.5	3
CHANGE	0.5	1	0.75	0.75
FINISH	2	2.75	2.25	3.75
ACQUIRED NEUROLOGICAL (12)				
START	1.91	2.16	1.58	2.75
CHANGE	0.54	0.75	0.79	0.37
FINISH	2.45	2.91	2.37	3.12
NEUROSURGERY (0)				
START				
CHANGE		NO PATIENTS		
FINISH				
OROFACIAL/NECK SURGERY (1)				
START	4	3	3	2
CHANGE	0	0	1	1
FINISH	4	3	4	3
PROGRESSIVE NEUROLOGICAL DISEASE (3)				
START	1.33	2.66	1.66	2.66
CHANGE	−0.66	−0.66	0	−1
FINISH	0.66	2	1.66	1.66
VOICE PATHOLOGY (16)				
START	2.65	3.03	3.31	2.68
CHANGE	0.93	0.9	1.06	1.25
FINISH	3.59	3.93	4.37	3.93
BURNS/PLASTICS (1)				
START	3	3	3	4
CHANGE	0	0.5	0	0
FINISH	3	3.5	3	4
DEVELOPMENTAL DELAY (113)				
START	2.15	2.59	2.56	3.12
CHANGE	0.38	0.43	0.47	0.28
FINISH	2.54	3.02	3.03	3.41
CEREBRAL PALSY (8)				
START	1.87	2.37	2.12	2.75
CHANGE	0	0.25	0.5	0.5
FINISH	1.87	2.62	2.62	3.25

(continued)

(continued)

ETIOLOGY	I	D	H	W
HEARING DISORDERS (0)				
START				
CHANGE		NO PATIENTS		
FINISH				
MULTIFACTORIAL (4)				
START	1.75	2.62	1.87	1.75
CHANGE	−0.37	−0.62	−0.25	0
FINISH	1.37	2	1.62	1.75
NOTHING ABNORMAL DETECTED (53)				
START	1.93	2.44	2.37	2.33
CHANGE	1.07	0.93	0.91	1.2
FINISH	3	3.37	3.29	3.53
SYNDROMES (21)				
START	2.14	2.45	2.23	2.66
CHANGE	0.14	0.38	0.35	0.33
FINISH	2.28	2.83	2.59	3
OTHERS (48)				
START	2.18	2.53	2.3	2.65
CHANGE	0.12	0.44	0.3	0.37
FINISH	2.31	2.97	2.6	3.03

APPENDIX M

Speech Therapy Outcomes
for Site 8

OVERALL VIEW
TOTAL NUMBER OF PATIENTS = 34

	I	D	H	W
START	2	2.17	2.38	3.02
CHANGE	0.58	0.91	0.85	0.63
FINISH	2.58	3.08	3.23	3.66

	% CHANGE IN I	NUMBER OF NO CHANGE	% CHANGE IN D	NUMBER OF NO CHANGE	% CHANGE IN H	NUMBER OF NO CHANGE	% CHANGE IN W	NUMBER OF NO CHANGE
ALL PATIENTS (34)	11.6	17	18.2	11	17	9	12.6	17

BY IMPAIRMENT

DISORDER	% CHANGE IN I	NUMBER OF NO CHANGE	% CHANGE IN D	NUMBER OF NO CHANGE	% CHANGE IN H	NUMBER OF NO CHANGE	% CHANGE IN W	NUMBER OF NO CHANGE
DISORDERS OF FLUENCY (9)	-3.2	7	6.6	5	5.4	4	10	3
DYSPHAGIA (4)	55	0	60	0	55	0	60	0
AUTISM (2)	20	0	30	0	30	0	20	1
DEVELOPMENTAL DISORDER OF LANGUAGE (3)	10	1	13.2	0	16.6	0	0	3
PHONOLOGICAL IMPAIRMENT (9)	6.6	5	6.6	5	8.8	4	0	7
LEARNING DISABILITY (7)	11.4	4	22.8	1	17	1	8.4	3

BY IMPAIRMENT

DISORDER	I	D	H	W
DISORDERS OF FLUENCY (7)				
START	2.55	2.55	2.66	2.55
CHANGE	−0.16	0.33	0.27	0.5
FINISH	2.38	2.88	2.94	3.05
DYSPHAGIA (4)				
START	1.5	1	1.25	1.5
CHANGE	2.75	3	2.75	3
FINISH	4.25	4	4	4.5
AUTISM (2)				
START	0.5	2	2	2
CHANGE	1	1.5	1.5	1
FINISH	1.5	3.5	3.5	3
DEVELOPMENTAL DISORDER OF LANGUAGE (3)				
START	2	2	2.33	3.66
CHANGE	0.5	0.66	0.83	0
FINISH	2.5	2.66	3.16	3.66
PHONOLOGICAL IMPAIRMENT (9)				
START	3	3.22	3.11	4
CHANGE	0.33	0.33	0.44	0
FINISH	3.33	3.55	3.55	4
LEARNING DISABILITY (7)				
START	0.74	1.14	1.85	3.28
CHANGE	0.57	1.14	0.85	0.42
FINISH	1.28	2.28	2.71	3.71

BY ETIOLOGY

ETIOLOGY	% CHANGE IN I	NUMBER OF NO CHANGE	% CHANGE IN D	NUMBER OF NO CHANGE	% CHANGE IN H	NUMBER OF NO CHANGE	% CHANGE IN W	NUMBER OF NO CHANGE
CARDIOVASCULAR DISEASE (3)	60	0	60	0	60	0	60	0
DEVELOPMENTAL DELAY (16)	10.6	7	15	5	11.4	5	5	9
NOTHING ABNORMAL DETECTED (13)	0	13	11.6	7	10	5	12.4	4
SYNDROMES (1)	0	1	0	1	20	0	20	0
OTHERS (1)	0	1	0	1	60	0	40	0

BY ETIOLOGY

ETIOLOGY	I	D	H	W
CARDIOVASCULAR DISEASE (3)				
START	1.33	1	0.66	1.33
CHANGE	3	3	3	3
FINISH	4.33	4	3.66	4.33
DEVELOPMENTAL DELAY (16)				
START	1.92	2.14	2.64	3.21
CHANGE	0.53	0.75	0.57	0.25
FINISH	2.46	2.89	3.21	3.46
NOTHING ABNORMAL DETECTED (13)				
START	2.33	2.41	2.58	2.75
CHANGE	0.16	0.58	0.5	0.62
FINISH	2.5	3	3.08	3.37
SYNDROMES (1)				
START	1	3	2	4
CHANGE	0	1	1	1
FINISH	1	4	3	5
OTHERS (1)				
START	0	0	1	5
CHANGE	0	2	3	0
FINISH	0	2	4	5

APPENDIX N

Future Requirements to Extend This Work

All studies come to an end before the work is completed. The main issues that remain to be addressed are:

Work to be undertaken

- Data collection over a longer period of time to allow analysis of therapy outcome information.
- Further interscorer reliability trials
    to confirm reliability results;
    to establish the amount of practice and training required.
- Further testing of validity.
- Development and amendment of scales required:
    Two measures of wellbeing/distress (one relating to family/caregiver and one relating to client);
    Two measures of impairment—to reflect cognitive changes as compared to speech and language changes (particularly for use with clients who are learning disabled/mentally retarded and clients who have head injuries).
- Investigation of the value of the agreement score.
- Investigation of the value of the prediction score.
- Investigation of use of this approach with other disciplines and as a multidisciplinary approach.
- Incorporating user/caregiver dimension with appropriate scale descriptors and procedures.